Your Brain and Body Answer Book

Publisher's Note

The editors of FC&A have taken careful measures to ensure the accuracy and usefulness of the information in this book. While every attempt was made to assure accuracy, some Web sites, addresses, telephone numbers, and other information may have changed since printing.

This book is intended for general information only. It does not constitute medical advice or practice. We cannot guarantee the safety or effectiveness of any treatment or advice mentioned. Readers are urged to consult with their health care professionals and get their approval before undertaking therapies suggested by information in this book, keeping in mind that errors in the text may occur as in all publications and that new findings may supersede older information.

"I am your Creator. You were in my care even before you were born."
Isaiah 44:2a

Your Brain and Body Answer Book and all material contained therein copyright © 2011 by FC&A Publishing. All rights reserved. Printed in the United States of America.

FC&A Medical Publishing®
103 Clover Green
Peachtree City, GA 30269

Produced by the staff of FC&A

ISBN 978-1-935574-15-6

Table of Contents

Age-related macular degeneration

center blind spot • difficulty in low light
• blurriness • dulled colors

Good vision means you're better at navigating through your world, avoiding bumps, falls, and accidents. If you can see well, it's easier to take part in life. There are fewer difficulties in exercising, cooking healthy meals, taking medications, engaging your mind, and staying independent. And how important is it to avoid the huge emotional impact of vision loss — depression, anxiety, and stress? For all these reasons, taking care of your eyes should be priority one, yet only 10 percent of seniors believe they are at risk of eye disease.

Age-related macular degeneration (AMD), the leading cause of blindness in people over age 60 in the United States, is expected to affect 18 million people by the year 2050. It's a sneaky condition, developing slowly and painlessly over a number of years. The symptoms can include:

- a blind or blurred spot in the center of your vision

- the need for more light to read or do close work

- difficulty adapting to low light

- overall blurriness

- decreased intensity or brightness of colors

- difficulty recognizing faces

The term itself, macular degeneration, explains the process of this disease. The macula is a small area at the back of your eye in the center of your retina. It is responsible for providing color and detail to your central vision. As you read, for instance, light is focused on your macula where millions of light-sensing cells called photoreceptors change the light into nerve signals. These travel along your optic nerve to your brain where you interpret them as words. When the photoreceptors in your macula are damaged, or degenerate, you lose this important central vision.

There are two kinds of macular degeneration, wet and dry, with most people — 90 percent of those suffering from AMD — having dry. The difference lies in how the macula is damaged.

Researchers are intrigued by an association between eye disease and problems with thinking and memory. In a study of over 2,000 seniors, those who scored in the lowest 25 percent on a standardized cognition test were twice as likely to have early AMD. The exact relationship is still under debate, but the warning is not — if you have either condition, dementia or AMD, get screened for the other one.

- Dry AMD. With dry macular degeneration, yellow-white waste deposits, called drusen, accumulate in the tissue beneath the macula. These deposits interfere with the photoreceptors, causing them to deteriorate. Vision loss occurs very gradually, may not occur in both eyes, and may never result in total blindness. At any time, the dry form can turn into the wet form.

- Wet AMD. Wet macular degeneration means abnormal blood vessels have grown and begun to leak under the macula. This scars the retina and changes the position of the macula, distorting and destroying your central vision. The wet form of AMD is a leading cause of irreversible blindness.

Age is the major risk factor for AMD, with the threat jumping to 30 percent if you're over age 75. But there are other issues that can affect your odds. You are more likely to develop AMD if you're white; female; a smoker; have a relative with the condition; have light blue or green eyes; have uncontrolled high blood pressure; have high blood levels of C-reactive protein, a chemical marker of inflammation; or are obese. There's no cure for AMD, so prevention is critical.

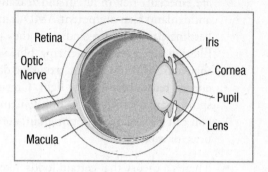

Retina
Optic Nerve
Macula
Iris
Cornea
Pupil
Lens

5 tactics to fight age-related macular degeneration

Eat like a Greek. No one really wants to go on a diet, even if it means saving your eyesight. So don't think of the Mediterranean diet as a diet, think of it as a fun, new way of looking at the foods you already eat.

- Your retina is teeming with omega-3 fatty acids. These help keep the cells there healthy and strong, able to fight off inflammation and death from oxidation. Researchers have studied people who eat omega-3-rich foods and found they really are protected against age-related macular degeneration (AMD). In fact, eating fish once a week cuts your risk by 40 percent. Eat it three times a week and you've reduced it by 75 percent. Fish like salmon and mackerel are great sources of omega-3 fatty acids, but olive oil and nuts like pecans, hazelnuts, and macadamias are also super ways to get this important fatty acid.

- Brightly colored fruits and vegetables are the backbone of the Mediterranean diet, and a powerhouse when it comes to eye health. They are brimming with antioxidants, like zinc and vitamins C and E, that safeguard the all-important photoreceptor cells in your macula. Yellow and green produce are especially rich in lutein and zeaxanthin, two specific antioxidants that are potent AMD fighters. In addition to battling damage from oxidation, they protect your retina by filtering dangerous high-energy, blue wavelengths of light that cause 100 times more oxidative damage than low-energy, red wavelengths of light. Green leafy vegetables like spinach are terrific sources of lutein and zeaxanthin, but you can also load up on pumpkin, corn, squash, broccoli, peas, or asparagus.

- There's a theory that certain foods, like white bread and potatoes, cause your blood sugar — or glucose — to spike. A sudden rush of glucose means more than usual floods into your cells. This can cause a host of problems, but one is damage to the delicate components in your eye. Foods that cause this kind of spike are considered to have a high Glycemic Index (GI). Others, low-GI foods, produce a more gradual increase in blood sugar. Complex carbohydrates, like fiber-rich fruits and vegetables and whole grains, are low-GI. Research out of Australia showed eating low-GI foods, especially cereal fiber such as oatmeal, can protect you from AMD, cutting your risk by one-third.

- Following the Mediterranean diet means eating fresh, whole foods and avoiding fast foods and processed, pre-packaged items. By doing this, you're avoiding trans fat. This unhealthy fat raises bad cholesterol levels and increases inflammation, damaging the blood vessels in your eyes just as it damages blood vessels elsewhere in your body. People with a lot of trans fats in their diet are more likely to develop AMD.

Drink deeply of D. Top off your new healthy eating plan with a big glass of vitamin D-fortified milk and see your way to a brighter future. Because of its anti-inflammatory properties, vitamin D fights the process that creates drusen beneath your macula. Of course, you can get vitamin D from a number of foods and even from supplements, but since milk is such an important part of a nutritious diet for many reasons, why not join the milk crew?

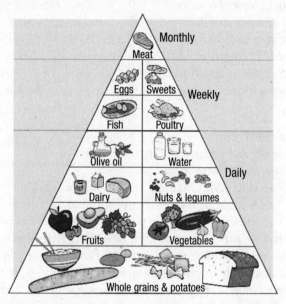

Mediterranean Diet: an eating plan that can save your vision

Take three B's to ease eye disease. A trio of B vitamins may keep your eyesight keen in a couple of ways. First, folic acid and vitamins B6 and B12 break down and eliminate homocysteine from your body. This naturally occurring amino acid damages the lining of your blood vessels and increases your risk of blood clots. Also, these same three B's can act as antioxidants, protecting the fragile photoreceptors in your eyes. Women who took B supplements daily — 2.5 milligrams (mg) of folic acid, 50 mg of vitamin B6, and 1 mg of vitamin B12 — for seven years were up to 40 percent less likely to develop AMD. Ask your doctor if B vitamin supplements are a smart choice for you.

Run away from AMD. If you're a runner, think about adding a few extra steps to your regular program. Bump your average jog up to at least two miles a day and you've more than doubled your protection against AMD compared to running a mile or less. And if you're not a runner, consider starting.

Test your blood. Carry one specific gene, and you're an astounding 700 percent more

likely to develop AMD than the average person. This one variation in your DNA could be responsible for forming the harmful drusen in your eye and for encouraging the abnormal growth of blood vessels that are part of the wet form of AMD. Drugs that can target this gene could be the hope of the future. In the meantime, ask your doctor about blood testing for gene typing, especially if you have a family history of AMD. Knowing your risk means you can take precautions now.

Amsler grid with normal vision

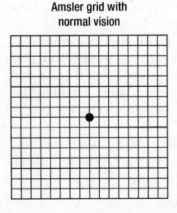

Amsler grid seen by someone with AMD

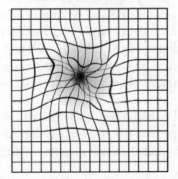

2 surprising ways to decrease the danger

There are two things you should never do if you want to cut the threat of developing AMD. First, never go outside without sunglasses. You'll not only look good, but you'll protect your peepers from the sun's harmful rays. Experts believe ultraviolet light causes damage to the pigment cells in your retina.

And don't take beta carotene supplements. Studies show people who boosted their beta carotene intake with pills had a higher risk of developing AMD.

Alpha-lipoic acid

improves memory • stimulates learning • controls blood sugar • soothes nerve pain • lowers trigylcerides • boosts metabolism • protects your vision

It sounds so tempting. Just pop a pill and boost your brainpower. It also sounds too good to be true. But in the case of alpha-lipoic acid, the results just might match the hype. This little-known but powerful supplement can repair your mental Rolodex. Research shows you'll be able to recall names instantly and regain your confidence.

Alpha-lipoic acid, a naturally occurring compound, has tremendous antioxidant powers. Unlike most antioxidants, it works in both water and fat. It may even help regenerate other antioxidants that have been used up. Another benefit is its positive effect on mitochondria, your cells' tiny powerhouses that burn food for energy.

This important coenzyme is synthesized in your body. You also can get it from some foods, including spinach, broccoli, yeast, tomatoes, peas, brussels sprouts, and organ meats, like liver. But to get enough of this sulfur-containing fatty acid to make a difference, you probably need supplements.

Studies suggest alpha-lipoic acid boosts metabolism, lowers triglycerides, fights diabetes and its complications, and it may help with other conditions, including glaucoma, multiple sclerosis, and burning mouth syndrome. Yet its effect on your brain could be its best feature. Find out how your brain can benefit from this super supplement.

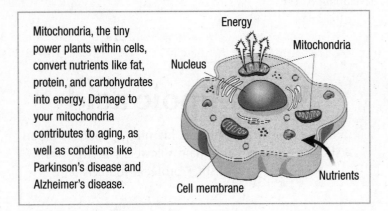

Mitochondria, the tiny power plants within cells, convert nutrients like fat, protein, and carbohydrates into energy. Damage to your mitochondria contributes to aging, as well as conditions like Parkinson's disease and Alzheimer's disease.

3 ways alpha-lipoic acid keeps you sharp

Maximizes your memory. A decline in mental sharpness often comes with age. So does the decay of mitochondria, your cells' energy factories. This decay has been linked to brain aging and diseases like Alzheimer's and Parkinson's. Luckily, alpha-lipoic acid can help solve both problems.

Several studies found that alpha-lipoic acid improved mental function, learning, and memory in old mice. The outlook for people is promising, too. One small study of people with

Alzheimer's and similar forms of dementia found that taking 600 milligrams of alpha-lipoic acid a day for a year stabilized their mental function.

Scientists have a few possible explanations for alpha-lipoic acid's brain-boosting powers.

- It improves memory-related signaling pathways.

- It reduces oxidative stress. Not only does alpha-lipoic acid neutralize harmful free radicals, it regenerates other anti-oxidants — which give themselves up, like kamikaze pilots, to stabilize free radicals — so they can do the same thing again. It also prevents metals like iron and copper from oxidizing and causing damage.

- It improves mitochondrial function. Alpha-lipoic acid protects mitochondria from oxidative damage, helps ward off the degeneration of brain cells, and even stimulates the production of new mitochondria.

Like a good employee, alpha-lipoic acid works well with others. Studies suggest that combining alpha-lipoic acid with other supplements, such as carnitine or coenzyme Q10, may lead to even better results. Animals given a combination of carnitine and alpha-lipoic acid had more energy and performed better on tests of learning and memory.

Defeats diabetes. Diabetes endangers more than your blood sugar levels. It goes hand-in-hand with obesity and heart problems. All of these conditions can negatively affect your brain.

Alpha-lipoic acid has shown promise in treating diabetes and its complications. Many small studies indicate alpha-lipoic acid may lower blood sugar levels in

> Most cells in your body contain between 500 and 2,000 mitochondria.

people with type 2 diabetes. In other studies, alpha-lipoic acid improved insulin sensitivity by 50 percent if taken intravenously and 25 percent if taken orally. It may also improve long-term blood sugar control, but more research is needed.

Here's another eye-opening tidbit about alpha-lipoic acid. It may help fight cataracts and glaucoma, vision problems that often affect older people.

Studies show that alpha-lipoic acid, whether taken intravenously or orally, improves the symptoms of diabetic neuropathy, or nerve damage, from continuously high blood sugar. In one study, people who took alpha-lipoic acid in doses ranging from 600 to 1,800 mg a day for five weeks experienced fewer symptoms, including less burning and stabbing pain.

Although there is some evidence alpha-lipoic acid may help, diabetes is a serious condition. Talk with your doctor before trying any alternative remedies, including supplements.

Tackles triglycerides. Like high cholesterol, triglycerides can put your health at risk. High levels of these lipids, or fats, in your blood can lead to obesity, diabetes, and heart disease. What's good for your heart and waistline is also good for your brain, so lowering triglycerides is a smart move.

Recent studies of lab rats found that alpha-lipoic acid lowered triglycerides by up to 60 percent. It worked by thwarting the synthesis of triglycerides in the liver and by whisking triglycerides out of the bloodstream. Scientists point out that alpha-lipoic acid works differently from triglyceride-lowering drugs, which often come with unwanted side effects, but it may be just as effective.

While it's not yet clear if alpha-lipoic acid has the same effect on people, it could be a promising new way to prevent or treat high triglyceride levels.

How to find the perfect mix

Alpha-lipoic acid comes in a variety of forms and pill strengths. The most common form on the market is a mixed form, or racemic, consisting of equal parts R (natural) and S (synthetic) isomers. This is also the form of alpha-lipoic acid used in most clinical trials.

You can also find supplements containing just the natural, R-isomer form, which animal studies suggest may be more effective at improving insulin sensitivity. But it's also more expensive than the racemic form.

To treat conditions like diabetes and its complications, the typical dosage is 600 to 1,200 milligrams (mg) a day divided into three equal doses. Experts say it's safe up to 1,800 mg. For generally healthy people, recommendations range from 200 to 400 mg a day to as little as 20 to 50 mg a day.

Take alpha-lipoic acid supplements on an empty stomach, either one hour before or two hours after eating, to maximize its impact.

Sound supplement strategies

Supplements aren't always what they seem. Because dietary supplements are not strictly regulated by the FDA, consumers have more choices — but less protection. That means less certainty that a product contains what it claims to contain.

Play it safe and buy supplements only from reputable sources. Also keep in mind that "natural" doesn't always mean "safe." Some dietary supplements may dangerously interact with prescription or over-the-counter drugs as well as other supplements.

Alpha-lipoic acid comes with its own specific concerns. Possible side effects include skin rash, hives, or itching. If you take medication for diabetes, you may need to adjust the dosage because of alpha-lipoic acid's beneficial effect on blood sugar. At high doses, alpha-lipoic acid may cause stomach pain, nausea, vomiting, dizziness, and headache.

Like any supplement, alpha-lipoic acid should only be taken after consulting your doctor.

Alzheimer's disease

forgetfulness • difficulty concentrating • speech problems
• confusion • depression • impaired judgment
• movement problems • behavior changes

Alzheimer's disease (AD) is not a normal part of aging. It is a serious disease with serious consequences, but there is a vast difference between minor memory problems you may experience as you age and this condition. Because of the devastating — and fatal — nature of AD, many people react out of fear. But the more information you have, the better equipped you'll be to confront AD if it touches your life.

Dementia, first of all, is a misunderstood term. Many people think Alzheimer's and dementia are completely different conditions. There are actually several different kinds of dementia — Alzheimer's is the most common, affecting more than 5 million Americans.

You are said to have dementia if a condition or disease has damaged your brain cells to the point you've lost memory and other mental abilities. People with dementia can suffer from personality changes, have difficulty speaking, problems walking, trouble thinking clearly, experience a decline in judgment, and face a host of other issues that interfere with daily life.

Read about the other types of dementia later in this chapter, and look for specific chapters that discuss some types of dementia in more detail.

A healthy brain sends information between billions of nerve cells, building thoughts, memories, and skills. With Alzheimer's, these nerve cells, or neurons, don't function properly and eventually die. This causes the parts of your brain in charge of memory, thinking, and behavior to deteriorate. Since AD is a progressive disease, the brain damage and its effects gradually expand and worsen.

> More than 70 percent of people with newly diagnosed Alzheimer's disease choose not to receive treatment the first year.

Right now, experts don't know what causes AD, and it's impossible to positively diagnose it without an autopsy. If you could look inside the brain of someone with AD, you'd always see two brain abnormalities, amyloid plaques and neurofibrillary tangles. Doctors don't know if these cause AD or if they are a result of the condition.

- Plaques and clumps. Beta-amyloid is a protein your brain's nerve cells need to pass on information. Sometimes, for unknown reasons, sticky clumps of beta-amyloid float between neurons or attach to pieces of damaged nerve cells and other proteins, building up into plaques.

- Tangles. Your brain cells have a complex transportation system called microtubules that deliver nutrients. A protein called tau normally helps support these microtubules, but in people with Alzheimer's, tau becomes damaged and twisted into threads that destroy the microtubules. These threads are called neurofibrillary tangles.

Plaques, clumps, and tangles mean neurons lose connection with each other. When they can't communicate, they die and brain tissue shrinks.

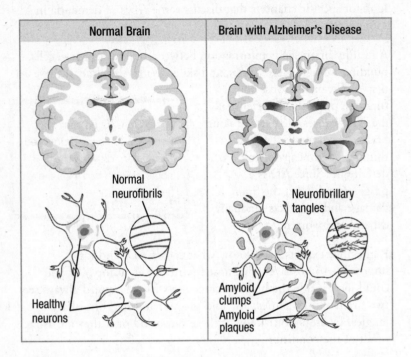

Normal Brain	Brain with Alzheimer's Disease

Normal neurofibrils

Neurofibrillary tangles

Amyloid clumps

Amyloid plaques

Healthy neurons

Test early to get a jump on treatment. A diagnosis of AD by autopsy is conclusive but not helpful in the here and now. That's why experts put a lot of faith in what they call a clinical diagnosis. This involves ruling out other conditions, gathering a medical history, and performing a variety of mental exams and interviews. Diagnosing AD as early as possible means:

- you can start drug treatment in the early stages of the disease, which may slow down the mental and physical decline.

- family members can begin to plan for the future in practical, financial, and legal ways.

- participating in a clinical trial of experimental drugs or treatments is an option.

Talk to your doctor about tests that might be helpful for you or a loved one.

Get smart on little-known symptoms. You might be surprised at some of the early signs of Alzheimer's.

- Loss of smell. It's common to lose your sense of smell years before you show other symptoms of AD. Researchers found that people who couldn't recognize more than two out of 10 common scents — like smoke, leather, and lemon — were almost five times more likely to be eventually diagnosed with AD than those who did better on the "sniff test."

- Rapid weight loss. Seniors who rapidly lost weight were almost three times more likely to develop dementia than those who lost weight more slowly. Experts believe early stages of the disease can cause difficulty eating or a general loss of interest in food or cooking.

- Decline in financial skills. In one four-year study at the University of Alabama, losing financial skills, like the ability to pay bills and manage a bank statement, showed up a year before an AD diagnosis.

- Trouble evaluating, thinking, and understanding. These skills start disappearing years before memory loss. Things like reading a map and completing a jigsaw puzzle require

An aspirin a day may not keep Alzheimer's away. For every study published showing nonsteroidal anti-inflammatory drugs (NSAIDs) like ibuprofen, naproxen, and aspirin reduce Alzheimer's risk, there's a report of NSAID use increasing risk. Ask your doctor if NSAIDs are a smart therapy for you.

you to recognize distances between objects, a skill that, in a University of Kansas study, declined three years before a clinical diagnosis of AD.

- Increase in "senior moments." Do you lose your train of thought or find yourself staring off into space? In a recent study, older folks who experienced at least three different symptoms of mental lapses like these were four and a half times more likely to be diagnosed with Alzheimer's.

Stages of Alzheimer's Disease	
Stage 1: No impairment	normal
Stage 2: Very mild decline	memory issues are not noticeable to others
Stage 3: Mild decline	a medical interview may identify difficulties; others notice problems
Stage 4: Moderate decline	mild or early-stage AD can be diagnosed; individuals are unable to perform complex tasks
Stage 5: Moderately severe decline	major memory and functioning problems make daily assistance necessary
Stage 6: Severe decline	mid-stage AD; full-time care may be needed due to significant memory, behavior, and personality changes
Stage 7: Very severe decline	late-stage AD; there is no response to the environment; individuals become unable to speak or control movement

Don't stress. Some things you just can't change — like three major risk factors for Alzheimer's.

- Genetics. Early-onset Alzheimer's, a rare form of the disease, usually runs in families, but experts are also looking at a specific gene, apolipoprotein E (ApoE), that may be linked to the more common late-onset Alzheimer's. Carrying this gene means you have a higher risk of developing Alzheimer's disease, not that you will definitely develop it.

- Age. Although AD is not a normal part of aging, age is the greatest risk factor — 96 percent of Americans with AD are age 65 or older.

- Gender. More women than men develop Alzheimer's. This may be because women tend to live longer.

Stress can affect your brain and mental abilities, so don't waste time worrying about these risk factors. Instead, think about the things you can change. Take charge of certain health conditions and you may be able to slow or stop AD's development.

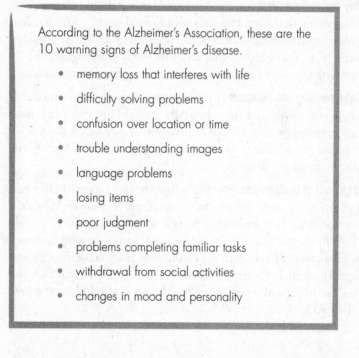

According to the Alzheimer's Association, these are the 10 warning signs of Alzheimer's disease.

- memory loss that interferes with life
- difficulty solving problems
- confusion over location or time
- trouble understanding images
- language problems
- losing items
- poor judgment
- problems completing familiar tasks
- withdrawal from social activities
- changes in mood and personality

5 tactics that fight Alzheimer's disease

Love your heart. If it's good for your heart, it's good for your brain. Multiple studies have shown high blood pressure, high cholesterol, and even diabetes — especially in middle age — increase your risk of developing Alzheimer's disease (AD) when you're older. Fight these conditions by controlling your weight, following a heart-smart diet, and exercising regularly.

Avoid a head injury. A blow to the head increases the chance you'll develop AD or another form of dementia. If you lose consciousness, experts say your risk of AD is almost 10 times higher. Fall-proof your home; wear good-fitting, supportive shoes; improve your balance with exercise; and ask your doctor if you are taking any medications that could be making you dizzy.

Stay mentally active. Engaging in hobbies, entertainment, or occupations that stimulate your mind could mean you're less likely to develop AD. Unfortunately, the opposite is also true. Long hours spent doing things that aren't mentally challenging, like watching television, are associated with a higher risk of dementia.

Make healthy life choices. Don't smoke, drink alcohol in moderation if you drink, and stay physically active. This way, you'll not only help your entire cardiovascular system stay healthy, you'll stimulate your brain to produce more neurons, blood vessels, and communication channels.

Eat to boost brainpower. Specific nutrients, like omega-3 fatty acids, B vitamins, or antioxidants, may contribute to a lower AD risk. But health professionals want you to understand a varied diet of whole foods gives your brain the best protection, possibly because of an interaction of nutrients. An eating plan like the Mediterranean diet, which includes fruits, vegetables, whole grains, and fish, is ideal for heart and whole-body health and is also linked to a lower risk of AD.

Defining dementia:
6 types you may not know

Vascular dementia. This second most common type of dementia is caused by blockages or leaks in blood vessels that decrease blood flow to your brain. High blood pressure, high cholesterol, and diabetes often cause the blood vessel damage behind vascular dementia.

Dementia with Lewy bodies. Lewy bodies are abnormal deposits of a specific protein — alpha-synuclein protein — that accumulate inside neurons in areas of your brain controlling memory and movement. There's no known prevention, treatment, or cure.

Parkinson's disease (PD). The main feature of PD is a loss of dopamine, a key neurotransmitter that affects movement, coordination, and information processing.

Frontotemporal dementia. This term includes three different disorders, all affecting a specific area of your brain controlling personality, behavior, and language. It's often mistaken for psychiatric disorders, Alzheimer's disease, or Parkinson's. There's no treatment or cure, but you can manage the symptoms with lifestyle changes and medications.

Creutzfeldt-Jakob disease (CJD). CJD belongs to a family of human and animal diseases known as the transmissible spongiform encephalopathies, which cause microscopic holes in your brain. This rare disorder triggers memory and behavior changes, as well as vision and coordination problems. There is no treatment or cure.

Normal pressure hydrocephalus (NPH). When the normal flow of fluid in your brain and spinal cord is blocked — due to infection, a tumor, surgery complications, a blow to the head, or an unknown cause — it builds up and puts pressure on your brain. The symptoms are so similar to other types of dementia that NPH is often misdiagnosed or treated improperly. This is particularly tragic since many people can recover completely once a shunt is placed in their brain to drain the excess fluid.

Ginkgo a no-go for dementia

The largest-ever study of ginkgo biloba for memory says the herb is a flop. More than 3,000 seniors were followed for six years — half took 120 milligrams of ginkgo extract twice daily, half took a placebo. Numerous tests showed no difference in mental decline between the two groups.

The fact it doesn't do much good for your memory is less alarming than concerns it could increase your risk of stroke. While it's well-known ginkgo has a blood-thinning effect and can increase your risk of bleeding, new evidence suggests it could be linked to a higher incidence of non-hemorrhagic stroke, the kind caused by a blocked blood vessel. In addition, those in the study with existing heart disease taking ginkgo were 56 percent more likely to develop dementia than those with heart disease taking the placebo.

> The Alzheimer's Association says aggressive medical treatment for people with advanced dementia is rarely successful and can speed up physical and mental decline. They suggest palliative care as an alternative. This type of treatment is designed to relieve symptoms rather than cure the disease.

Experts believe the ginkgo-heart link deserves more investigation. In the meantime, if you have heart disease, have a serious discussion with your doctor before taking ginkgo supplements.

Self-tests mean early diagnosis

They're here — quick and accurate tests that screen for Alzheimer's disease and other types of dementia. The Test Your Memory (TYM) contains tasks that evaluate 10 kinds of mental skills. In a recent study, the TYM correctly identified 93 percent of AD cases.

The Self-Administered Gerocognitive Examination is a four-page written test that, in new research, proves to be 80 percent accurate in recognizing early memory and thinking problems. Your doctor should be able to provide either of these tests in his office.

Aromatherapy

eases anxiety • boosts mood • soothes
muscle pain • relieves headaches • keeps you alert
• helps you sleep • curbs appetite

One little whiff and you're instantly connected to a feeling or a memory. Odors can cause your body to respond in many ways. The intriguing relationship between your nose and your brain has scientists sniffing and spritzing in an attempt to understand aromatherapy, the use of natural, fragrant plant oils for better health. But to begin with, you must unravel that most wonderful of the five senses — smell.

The purpose of your nose is to warm and clean the air you breathe in. Without your sense of smell, not only would you miss the lovely aroma of fresh-brewed coffee, you couldn't smell the smoke of a fire or tell if your food was spoiled.

The most direct way inhaled scents enter your body is through the mucous membranes in your nose. The molecules are so small they are easily absorbed and quickly make their way into your

> When used in massage, essential oils are absorbed through your skin as well as inhaled. They soak through your tissues and enter your bloodstream, where they are carried to all the organs and systems of your body.

bloodstream. They circulate throughout your body and, many people believe, directly affect specific internal organs like your intestines, kidneys, and lungs. Another, more complex, journey better explains the connection between scents and your brain.

At the very top of your nasal cavity is a patch of millions of specialized cells called the olfactory epithelium. These receptors are sensitive to odor molecules in the air. When an odor stimulates a receptor cell, it sends an electrical impulse to a group of structures in your brain called the limbic system.

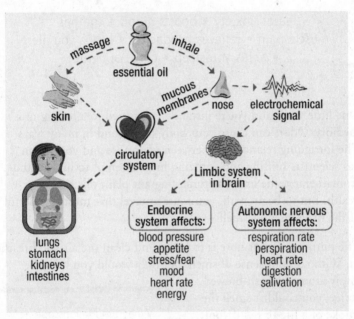

These specific parts of your brain are in charge of smell, as well as certain moods and feelings. In fact, the limbic system is sometimes considered the emotional center of your brain. No wonder smell and emotions are so closely linked. Experts think there are two ways scent can impact your mood and behavior.

The first time you smell a new scent, your brain links it to something going on around you or the way you feel at that moment. This is especially true for intense situations. Your brain builds a connection between that smell and a memory. The next time you encounter that scent, your brain pulls up the connection and you feel that way again.

Perhaps your first date was at a county fair and now the smell of cotton candy makes you feel excitedly happy. Someone else had a scary ride on a roller coaster at the fair and the smell of cotton candy makes them feel queasy. Some researchers call this process autobiographical odor memory.

Another school of thought is that this relationship is purely chemical. Your limbic system connects to automatic functions like breathing and circulation, as well as to your endocrine system, which is in charge of hormones. When an odor triggers an electrical signal to your brain, any number of neurotransmitters could fire up, affecting things like your heart rate or your fight-or-flight response.

> Looking for a certified aromatherapist? Go online at *www.aromatherapycouncil.org* and search for one in your area. There are 19 schools that offer programs approved by the National Association for Holistic Aromatherapy. If you want to learn more about accreditation, visit the website for the Alliance of International Aromatherapists at *www.alliance-aromatherapists.org.*

Although random scents can bring up memories and make you feel a certain way, using aromas to purposefully create a response requires the use of essential oils. By crushing or distilling the leaves, peel, or bark of certain plants, experts can extract an oil filled with its fragrance. When this is done naturally, without chemicals, it's called an essential oil. How an essential oil smells and is used by your body varies based on its chemical structure.

Understanding and manipulating the link between specific odors and a controlled behavior is something scientists are still working on. Aromatherapy can improve some health conditions, but there's no evidence it can prevent or cure any major illness.

5 ways aromatherapy keeps you sharp

Calms you down and cheers you up. A scent you associate with a happy memory can recreate that original feeling of well-being. You'll find it's almost impossible to be stressed or depressed at the same time you're feeling happy. So nose out whatever special, comforting aroma triggers your feel-good memories, and let it boost your mood.

For a more clinical explanation, consider that to shrug off tension, anxiety, and depression, you need to calm your breathing, stabilize your heart rate and blood pressure, and rein in the amount of the stress hormone, cortisol, pouring into your bloodstream. All this is controlled by your endocrine and autonomic nervous systems, which get their marching orders from the limbic system in your brain.

There's a revolutionary new product in town, and it sure smells good. Nasal SoftStrips are FDA-approved, over-the-counter strips instilled with either peppermint, to curb your appetite, or lavender, to help you de-stress and relax. Simply fit a strip around the bottom of your nose and breathe deeply for a few minutes.

If the right scent triggers just the right signal from your nose to your limbic system, you've put the kibosh on all those underlying issues. For instance, the kitchen herb marjoram can relieve anxiety, lower high blood pressure by dilating your blood vessels, and help you rest.

Many studies on aromatherapy for stress, anxiety, and depression use massage as a way of introducing scents to your body. The results are often positive, but consider the possibility that the massage itself is improving your mood and relaxing away tension.

Soothes pain naturally. Just as certain smells can be so irritating they give you a headache, others can be so pleasing they make your pain go away. It's not just one component of an essential oil that does the job, but a complex mixture reaching your brain and triggering different responses. Some affect neurotransmitters like dopamine that are closely linked to processing pain, and others encourage the release of endorphins, which are your body's natural painkillers. Using an essential oil along with massage can be doubly helpful for muscle pain and even headaches.

Prevents brain drain. Certain odors are sharp enough to grab your attention, helping you to stay focused on the task at hand. Whether you're combating fatigue, trying to complete a task, or need to remember something, breathe in a scent known to stimulate your nervous system, like peppermint or cinnamon.

Helps you sleep like a baby. Scents that relax can be an important part of a successful bedtime routine. Quiet time, warm baths, gentle stretching, and deep breathing all calm your mind and your muscles. Factor in a scent, like lavender, that's proven to promote better quality sleep, and you're almost guaranteed to catch some shut-eye.

Controls your appetite. The smell of a delicious food triggers the memory of eating and enjoying that food and can instantly get your stomach juices flowing. Could the opposite be true? How wonderful to go on a "sniff" diet and watch those pounds melt away.

Your hypothalamus, an area of your brain the size of a cherry, controls hunger, and its opposite — satiety, or a feeling of fullness.

Scents that fire a string of chemical reactions can muzzle that hungry beast in your belly by telling your hypothalamus what to do. Scientists found this to be true with the smells of peppermint and grapefruit.

Anosmia is the loss of your sense of smell. Often, it is caused by sinus disease or infections that cause swelling within your nose, or polyps that block odors from reaching the olfactory area. Treating the infection or removing the polyps can return your sense of smell. Head trauma is a more serious, and often permanent, cause of anosmia.

	Stress	Depression	Insomnia	Fatigue/ Memory	Pain	Weight gain
basil		✔				
chamomile	✔	✔	✔			
cinnamon				✔		
citrus	✔	✔				
clary sage	✔	✔				
clove					✔	
eucalyptus	✔	✔		✔		
frankincense	✔				✔	
ginger					✔	
grapefruit						✔
jasmine	✔	✔				
juniper					✔	
lavender	✔	✔	✔		✔	
lemon	✔				✔	
marjoram	✔		✔		✔	
peppermint	✔			✔	✔	✔
rose	✔	✔			✔	
rosemary		✔		✔	✔	
sandalwood		✔				
ylang-ylang	✔	✔			✔	

Sweet-smelling strategies keep you safe

Essential oils are very concentrated, so be careful how you use them.

- Never swallow any unless specifically prescribed by your doctor.

- Before using any essential oil on your skin, dilute it in a carrier oil, such as almond, coconut, jojoba, or sunflower.

- Respect your allergies. If you're allergic to nuts, don't use carrier oils made from almonds or peanuts. If you have hay fever, you may react to inhaling chamomile.

- Keep bottles of essential oils out of direct light and tightly sealed. They can break down and become irritating.

> The average person can recognize up to 10,000 separate odors.

- Less is more. Start with just a bit of fragrance to see how you react. Scented commercial products, like diffusers, candles, bath salts, and lotions, may be all you need to reap the benefits.

Beta carotene

sweet potato • carrots • spinach • cantaloupe • mango • papaya

Poets have a tough time finding a word that rhymes with "orange." But you don't have to be a poet to appreciate the beauty of bright orange fruits and vegetables.

Beta carotene, the pigment that gives these foods their orange color, also gives you plenty of health benefits. And there are plenty of foods that provide beta carotene, the most common carotenoid. Carotenoids are pigments ranging from light yellow to reddish orange. Besides bright orange fruits and veggies, beta carotene is also found in dark green vegetables. The combination of the green pigment chlorophyll and orange beta carotene produces the dark green color.

Think of beta carotene as the plant form of vitamin A, which is found in animal products like liver, dairy, and eggs. In fact, your body converts beta carotene to vitamin A, or retinol. Like vitamin A, beta carotene acts as an antioxidant. It helps preserve your eyesight, strengthens your immune system, and fights cancer, heart disease, and other serious conditions.

1 baked sweet potato	16.8 mg*
1 cup cooked carrots	12.9 mg
1 cup cooked spinach	11.3 mg
1 cup cantaloupe	3.2 mg
1 mango	0.92 mg
1 papaya	0.84 mg

* milligrams

Thanks mostly to its antioxidant activity, beta carotene also does wonders for your brain. Read on to discover more about this orange superstar.

3 ways beta carotene keeps you sharp

Boosts memory. Remember to eat your carrots, and you'll remember much more. In a Swiss study of people ranging in age from 65 to 94, those with higher blood levels of beta carotene performed better on several memory tests. Researchers aren't sure exactly how beta carotene aids your memory, but eating more fruits and vegetables may give you an edge.

That's because the antioxidant powers of beta carotene may protect your brain from dementia. The Physicians Health Study II, which followed nearly 6,000 men age 65 or older, found that beta carotene supplements may guard against mental decline — but only with long-term use. Men who took beta carotene supplements for 15 years or more had slightly higher scores on memory tests, but those who took the supplements for three years or less showed no benefit. Although the differences were small, even very modest differences in memory can lead to big differences in the risk of developing dementia.

In lab tests, vitamin A helps control beta-amyloid buildup, which plays a role in the development of Alzheimer's disease. Antioxidants also help improve brain function.

A University of California, Los Angeles study determined that high blood levels of beta carotene may protect against mental decline in older people who carry a certain gene that makes them more susceptible to Alzheimer's disease. The Alzheimer's Association even recommends including dark colored vegetables and colorful fruits in your diet for protection. It's a simple step that helps you think more clearly as you age.

Defeats depression. Eating brightly colored fruits and vegetables may brighten your mood. A Japanese study found that older men who ate the most carotenoids had fewer symptoms of depression. Compared to those who got the least carotene in their diet, those with the highest intake had a 64 percent lower risk of having symptoms of depression. There were similar results among older women, but the results were not statistically significant.

Researchers point to carotenoids' antioxidant powers as a possible explanation. Carotenoids may protect your brain from oxidative stress, which contributes to major depression. Oxidative stress refers to the damage caused by the production of molecules called reactive oxygen species, which include free radicals. As an antioxidant, beta carotene helps neutralize these harmful substances.

Looking for more beta carotene? Try sweet peppers, apricots, grapefruit, squash, and watermelon. But don't forget dark leafy vegetables like collard, turnip, beet, and mustard greens, as well as kale. You can even get some beta carotene from broccoli, lettuce, peas, and brussels sprouts.

Safeguards your heart. When weighing a decision, you may sense a struggle between your heart and your brain. But when it comes to your health, they go hand-in-hand.

Many of the risk factors for heart disease also impact your brain. For example, people with bigger waists, more belly fat, and type 2 diabetes are also at greater risk for dementia. The common link is too much insulin. High blood pressure, which can lead to strokes, can also lead to dementia. It may cause a series of mini strokes, weaken the blood-brain barrier that guards your brain from toxins, or speed up the progression of Alzheimer's disease.

So when you take care of your heart, you're also protecting your brain. Luckily, beta carotene can help. As an antioxidant, it protects against DNA damage from oxidative stress, which can lead to cancer and heart disease. In a small Tufts University study, older women who took carotenoid supplements, including beta carotene, had less DNA damage in as little as 15 days.

Beta carotene may even keep your cholesterol under control. Lab tests show beta carotene and other carotenoids block cholesterol oxidation caused by free radicals. This could help prevent the thickening of your artery walls that occurs in atherosclerosis. In a French study, carrots reduced cholesterol absorption in rats.

Dutch researchers found that beta carotene may fight metabolic syndrome, a combination of four risk factors — high blood sugar, abdominal fat, high blood pressure, and high cholesterol — that boost your risk for heart disease, diabetes, and stroke.

Those with the highest intake of beta carotene had a 42 percent lower risk of metabolic syndrome compared to those with the lowest intake. More beta carotene was also associated with slimmer waists and smaller bellies.

Super strategies for the supermarket

Get the most out of beta carotene with these smart tips.

Eat a little fat. Fat is your friend — at least when it comes to beta carotene. Because beta carotene is fat-soluble, you need at least a little fat for your body to absorb it. That means ditching the fat-free salad dressing. A small Iowa State study found that you absorb virtually no beta carotene from salads with fat-free dressing. You get much more by using full-fat dressing than reduced-fat options.

Just make sure you pair your fruits and veggies with healthy fats, like monounsaturated fat from olive oil, nuts, and avocados. Try dipping your carrots in hummus for a healthy snack.

> Too much beta carotene, whether from food or supplements, may turn your skin yellow. It's an odd but harmless side effect.

Consider buying organic. Organic produce costs more, but it may be worth it. Some studies show you get nearly 50 percent more beta carotene from some organic fruits and vegetables compared to their conventionally grown counterparts. What's more, you also lessen your exposure to pesticides.

Be choosy. When choosing grapefruit, you're better off red. Red grapefruit, which contains more beta carotene than white grapefruit, also does a better job of scavenging dangerous free radicals and lowering triglycerides in your blood.

The danger of supplements

Foods containing beta carotene provide so many benefits researchers expected beta carotene supplements to work well, too. Instead, studies have shown some disturbing trends. Beta carotene supplements may boost the risk of some cancers, heart problems, and even death.

One large study found that smokers who took beta carotene supplements had an 18 percent greater incidence of lung cancer. Another major study was stopped early after researchers found that the participants taking beta carotene supplements were 46 percent more likely to die of lung cancer.

A Harvard study found that beta carotene supplements had no effect on the risk of heart attack, stroke, or death in women at risk for heart disease, while others show an increase in heart attack, stroke, and cardiovascular deaths. One Danish review of 47 studies found that people taking beta carotene supplements had a 7 percent higher risk of death from all causes.

Play it safe and get your beta carotene from a variety of delicious fruits and vegetables. Experts recommend aiming for 3 to 6 milligrams daily.

Getting enough vitamin A is easy as pie

You probably eat pumpkin pie only on Thanksgiving. Enjoy this holiday favorite more often to help protect your vision, your memory, and more. A slice of homemade pumpkin pie provides 7.4 milligrams of beta carotene and a whopping 249 percent of your daily vitamin A needs.

You need adequate amounts of vitamin A to ward off vision problems. Best of all, you don't need to bake a pie to reap the benefits of pumpkin. Cut down on the fat and calories by enjoying pumpkin in healthier ways. A side dish of mashed pumpkin with a sprinkle of cinnamon could be the best food you're not eating.

Brain aerobics

crossword puzzles • board games • creative writing
• a new skill or hobby • music or art class
• a second language • card games

Think of your brain as a muscle. Just like any other muscle in your body, you must follow the old adage of "use it or lose it." Give your brain its own trip to the gym and you could delay or slow the progress of Alzheimer's disease and other forms of dementia.

Years ago, experts thought each person was born with all the brain cells they would ever have. Then, not only did they learn you could form new cells throughout your life, but you could also change and rewire your brain based on knowledge and experience. So just as someone with little muscle tone in their arms and legs can exercise their way to a stronger and more fit body, you can work out your brain and enjoy sharper thinking.

Learn something new. Doing something you haven't done before means your brain must form new connections. Challenge yourself with different activities, both physical and mental, and your brain responds by changing and growing, becoming better, faster, and leaner.

There is no age limit and you can't rest on your laurels. Let's say you've mastered a complicated task or activity — like the numbers puzzle Sudoku. Or perhaps you're a whiz at the *New York Times* crossword. That means those neural pathways are built. Your brain doesn't have to work so hard anymore and you're actually in an intellectual rut. To get the real benefit of mental exercise, you've got to

> Choose your friends carefully. To stretch your mind, surround yourself with people who are dynamic and interesting and who can offer new ideas and perspectives.

constantly move on to something harder, challenging your brain with activities that are new and different.

Build up a reserve. It's quite possible you could have evidence of dementia inside your brain, but never suffer from the symptoms. That's because you've built up what is called a cognitive reserve. It's like a savings account for brainpower. Even if the funds in your checking account are dwindling, you can always call on this extra bit you've set aside for a rainy day. The more you work out your mind, the greater your cognitive reserve. And the more you have in reserve, the better able you are to defy the effects of aging.

In a review combining data from 29,000 people and 22 studies worldwide, experts discovered that those who built up a cognitive reserve by staying mentally active reduced their risk of Alzheimer's disease and other forms of dementia by nearly half. Here's more evidence.

- The Rush University Medical Center in Chicago found that mentally active seniors, with an average age of 80, were 2.6 times less likely to develop dementia than others.

- In the 5-year Bronx Aging Study, for every day seniors engaged in a brain-stimulating activity, they delayed the rapid memory loss linked to dementia by two months.

Not every mental exercise is equally beneficial. Decide if an activity will challenge your brain in one or more of these five critical areas:

visual-spatial skills	your ability to recognize and understand two-dimensional and three-dimensional figures
motor function	your ability to use and control your muscles
executive function	your ability to organize thoughts and activities, prioritize tasks, manage time efficiently, and make decisions
language	your ability to communicate
memory	your ability to recall information

4 brain aerobics that keep you sharp

Lifelong learning. Become a student for life. Just 15 minutes a day learning something unfamiliar means your brain is building new cells and communication pathways. While doing harder crossword puzzles or tackling more complicated recipes in the kitchen will stretch your current abilities, challenging yourself with something un-related is even better at building brainpower. For big benefits, have a go at something completely different from your existing strengths.

> Brain plasticity is defined as the brain's ability to change itself when challenged.

Say you play the piano. Learn the oboe. You'll have to use your hands differently, breathe in a special way, and even use a new posture. If you write well, try working with numbers or science. If you're an account-ant, take an art or dancing class to stimulate the other side of your brain. Learning another language is one more terrific way to build neural connections. To stay on top of your mental game now and in the years to come, never stop looking for new things to learn or new ways to engage in old activities.

Games and puzzles. Roll your lucky dice, deal a winning hand, or count out those points — however you play, you can be sure you're coming in first when it comes to brainpower. Games aren't just for kids anymore. While you're sharpening your pencil, you'll be sharpening your thinking skills and slashing your risk of dementia.

In the famous Bronx Aging Study, seniors who played board games several times a week cut their chances of developing dementia by an astounding 74 percent. Crossword puzzles four days out of seven cut their risk almost in half. Just be sure you choose something challenging and mix it up.

Reading. Of course, you read something every day. But amp it up and you'll make a deposit into your oh-so-important cognitive reserves. Choose material that makes you think or teaches you something new. Join a book club or reading group so you're forced to analyze and discuss what you've read. Look up unfamiliar words in the dictionary and mull over new ideas. Try an author or genre outside your comfort zone to add an element of change to the activity. All this builds vocabulary, memory, reading efficiency, and knowledge and can cut your risk of dementia.

Neurobics. Is there a rebel hidden inside of you? Ever dream of throwing tradition to the wind and doing things in a completely new and challenging way? Here's your chance, and you'll be giving your brain a workout at the same time.

That's the concept behind Neurobics, a term coined by Lawrence Katz, Professor of Neurobiology at Duke University Medical Center, and Manning Rubin, a writer in the communications and advertising business. Neurobics describes exercises designed to increase your brain's ability to stay fit, learn, and remember. To be considered a Neurobic exercise, it must:

- use one or more of your senses in a different way while you are participating in an ordinary activity.

- stand out from a normal activity because it's surprising, unusual, or fun.

- vary a routine in an unexpected way.

Want to keep your mind agile? Go on the Internet to *www.thinks.com* and try out some different games when you're tired of the crossword — they're especially designed to boost your memory and cognition.

Sudoku is the Japanese logic-based number placement puzzle that comes in many variations. You'll also find brainteasers, puzzle games, and word games. You can even do jigsaw puzzles or play chess, checkers, and Chinese checkers.

By changing how you do something, you change how you think about it, which physically changes your brain. Switching on little-used nerve pathways produces a kind of natural brain fertilizer that strengthens nerve connections, helping your brain stay young and fit. Katz and Rubin claim that everyday life is the Neurobic brain gym. That means you can engage in Neurobic exercises anywhere and at anytime. Here are some examples.

- If you are right-handed, brush your teeth with your left hand.

- Get dressed with your eyes closed.

- Completely rearrange your office.

- Select the correct change from your coin purse without looking.

- Listen to a completely new genre of music on the radio.

- Drive somewhere familiar using a totally new route.

For more information about Neurobics, visit their website at *www.neurobics.com*.

14 days to a better memory

A landmark study out of the University of California, Los Angeles showed you can fire up your brainpower in just two weeks. Researchers combined healthy lifestyle strategies into a four-step program, then, after 14 days, tested the participating seniors' mental skills, including memory. They found those on the program showed significant improvements. Here's how you can put this plan into action for yourself.

- Eat a healthy diet. Fuel your brain with five meals a day focusing on antioxidant-rich fruits and vegetables, whole grains, and omega-3 fatty acids.

- Engage in daily exercise. Strengthen your heart and avoid diseases that can impact brain health by walking briskly for 30 to 45 minutes a day.

- Reduce stress. Relax by stretching or deep breathing to reduce the amount of cortisol, a stress hormone that can shrink your brain's memory center.

- Train your memory. Mental exercises, like brainteasers and puzzles, challenge your brain to work harder and flourish.

Caffeine

coffee • energy drinks • tea
• colas • chocolate

Everyone knows at least one coffee fiend. It may even be you. Some labor over the bean selection, carefully grinding, meticulously brewing. Others prowl from coffeehouse to cafe, as if on the quest for the Holy Grail. Others don't care what it is as long as it's hot and strong. What is it about the lowly cup of joe that inspires such dedication?

It's mostly about the caffeine — a natural chemical that gives a boost of energy and brainpower. Coffee is just one way to get your kick, and over half of all Americans drink it every day. But don't forget the cola addicts. You can get anywhere from 30 to almost 50 milligrams of caffeine in one can.

8-oz. cup brewed coffee	133 mg*
8.3-oz. can Red Bull	80 mg
8-oz. cup brewed tea	53 mg
12-oz. can Diet Coke	47 mg
12-oz. can Pepsi	38 mg
1.45-oz. Hershey's Special Dark Chocolate Bar	31 mg

* milligrams

Caffeine is found naturally in coffee beans, tea leaves, cocoa beans, and kola nuts. Once you ingest it, it works much like a drug to stimulate your nervous system.

The good news is, getting about 100 to 200 milligrams of caffeine, the amount in the average cup of coffee or a couple of sodas, can make you feel more alert, relieve drowsiness, and improve your thinking.

6 ways caffeine keeps you sharp

Fine-tunes your focus. It's probably one of the reasons you drink coffee in the first place — to feel sharper, to react a little quicker, or to remember one more thing on your to-do list. You'll be happy to know it's more than just a feeling. Science is behind this 100 percent.

Caffeine is a stimulant. And that stimulatory effect is what makes you feel attentive and more focused in the short-term. You have extra neurons firing in your brain, and you've got adrenaline pumping through your system. The stress response in your body is triggered, so your senses are on high alert and your heart pushes blood and oxygen a little faster.

All this can be a good thing if you need a pick-me-up to help you hone your attention and focus. It can be a bad thing if it goes on too long. You'll read about the dangers of too much caffeine later.

Preserves your memories. Caffeine is also an anti-inflammatory and Alzheimer's disease (AD) is, in part, inflammation gone wrong. There's evidence that caffeine could delay AD and even protect against vascular dementia — memory loss and confusion from impaired blood flow to the brain. But it's groundbreaking animal research suggesting caffeine halts the formation of dangerous beta-amyloid protein that has scientists really excited.

One of the characteristics of AD is the accumulation of naturally occurring protein fragments between nerve cells in the brain.

Normally, these fragments are broken down and removed. In someone with AD, however, they accumulate and form destructive plaques. Caffeine keeps your body from making certain enzymes necessary to produce beta-amyloid. Not only is the caffeine protecting you against developing future memory problems, but it may someday reverse existing memory impairment.

When it comes down to balancing the possible benefits of caffeine against the dangers of overindulgence, scientists say there's a point of diminishing return. A little caffeine may not be enough to experience the brain-boosting benefits, but too much can cause side effects, like anxiety, headaches, and an irregular heartbeat. So what's the magic number?

Multiple studies show drinking four or more cups of caffeinated coffee a day means a lower risk of developing and dying from heart disease.

A group of researchers in Finland and Sweden say people who drink three to five cups of coffee a day are less likely to develop Alzheimer's disease or other forms of dementia. If you only drink one or two cups, you're not getting the same protection, and more than five a day is associated with side effects. In one four-year study, women — especially those 65 to 74 years old, and those who drank more than three cups every day — showed the most positive, memory-boosting effects.

Relaxes your arteries. You might be surprised if your doctor told you to go ahead and enjoy your favorite latte, even though you have high blood pressure. Doesn't caffeine make your blood pressure skyrocket? If you're a regular coffee drinker, you've developed at least a partial tolerance to the effects of caffeine on your blood pressure. If you indulge occasionally, you'll probably experience only a minor, temporary increase.

Although most people have heard caffeine described as a vasoconstrictor — meaning it narrows or constricts your blood vessels — when your body breaks down caffeine in the liver, it forms theobromine, a compound that causes your blood vessels to dilate. That's a good thing when your heart is having to work extra hard.

You may want to stick with coffee as a source of caffeine, because experts found that caffeinated colas are linked to a higher rate of high blood pressure.

Helps your heart. To protect your cholesterol levels, you can still "fill it to the rim," but you're going to have to get picky about your brewing techniques. Filtered coffee protects against the bad type of cholesterol, called LDL, but the boiled or unfiltered variety contains compounds that can actually increase LDL cholesterol levels. Instant coffee doesn't seem to have any effect one way or the other.

Arteries that are in good shape make it easier to pump blood and oxygen to your brain. When your arteries and blood vessels become stiff or clogged with cholesterol, your brain doesn't get enough oxygen. Brain cells begin to die and you experience problems like short-term memory loss.

Decreases your diabetes risk. Diabetes is bad news for your memory. Not only does it damage your blood vessels and hamper blood and oxygen flow to your brain, but spikes in blood sugar also damage brain cells. On the other hand, there's good news about caffeine and diabetes.

Whether you get your caffeine from green tea or coffee, you're lowering your risk of developing type 2 diabetes — especially if you're a long-time drinker. One cup of coffee a day reduces your risk by 13 percent, but four or more cups cuts it almost in half. If you already have diabetes, coffee will not make your diabetes worse or increase your risk of diabetic complications, assuming you don't load it with sugar or other unhealthy add-ons.

Caffeine interferes with your body's ability to absorb most vitamins and minerals. So drink your coffee and wait an hour to take your daily vitamin or calcium supplement.

Scientists say there are several possible explanations for caffeine's benefit.

- Caffeine decreases insulin sensitivity.

- More caffeine can mean less long-term weight gain, less dangerous belly fat, and a greater sense of fullness.

- It's possible that caffeine helps move glycogen — a storage form of glucose — out of your muscles to help keep blood sugar levels constant.

- Drinking coffee affects the amount of certain peptides you produce in your intestinal tract, which lowers glucose absorption in your small intestine.

Protects against Parkinson's. Memory loss, confusion, and slowed thinking are symptoms of Parkinson's disease (PD). Multiple studies show that daily coffee drinkers are at a lower risk of developing PD.

It all has to do with dopamine, a specific neurotransmitter, or chemical, used to carry messages between neurons. Dopamine is key in regulating working memory, and PD destroys dopamine-producing neurons. Caffeine, on the other hand, increases dopamine levels.

Experts are hopeful that caffeine has the potential to restore broken learning and memory processes in people with this illness.

The problem with labels

It would be nice to know what products contain caffeine and how much, whether you're trying to amp up your caffeine intake for more alertness or drop it down a notch to control the jitters. Unfortunately, the U.S. Food and Drug Administration doesn't make manufacturers list caffeine content on food labels. Some companies list it because they want you to know you're getting a kick-start jolt of this stimulant.

Take, for instance, Sumseeds, marketed as Energized Sunflower Seeds. These tasty little tidbits are "infused" with caffeine and other things. A single-serve, 1.75-ounce bag delivers a whopping 140 milligrams of caffeine. That's about equal to the caffeine content of two espressos.

An independent laboratory reviewed 53 products including a variety of supplements. They found if you took the products as directed, you could ingest anywhere from 1 to 829 milligrams of caffeine in one day. That's as much as you'd get in up to eight cups of coffee. But here's the real kicker — 25 of the products didn't even list caffeine as an ingredient.

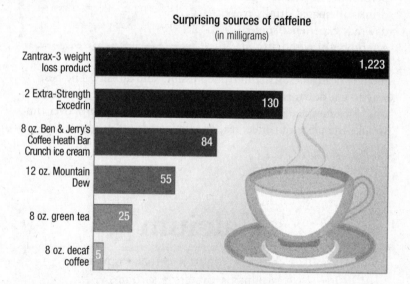

Surprising sources of caffeine
(in milligrams)

Source	Milligrams
Zantrax-3 weight loss product	1,223
2 Extra-Strength Excedrin	130
8 oz. Ben & Jerry's Coffee Heath Bar Crunch ice cream	84
12 oz. Mountain Dew	55
8 oz. green tea	25
8 oz. decaf coffee	5

Calming news about caffeine withdrawal

Caffeine is a drug. And like any other drug it carries inherent dangers. The most alarming are the effects of overdose. Get too much caffeine and you could feel everything from nausea to irritability to abnormal heart rhythms.

The problem is every person is different, and many factors influence how much caffeine is safe and healthy for you — including your metabolism rate, your body's caffeine tolerance, and underlying medical conditions.

If you feel the caffeine in your life is starting to negatively influence your health, consider cutting back. But if you've been a true caffeine junkie, do this carefully. Scientists say about half of the 80 to 90 percent of Americans who drink caffeinated drinks every day may experience some symptoms of withdrawal if they stop suddenly. These can include headaches, irritability, depression, and anxiety. The best way to cut down is gradually — drink a half-cup instead of a full one, for example, and introduce decaffeinated substitutes over time to take the place of coffee, tea, or caffeinated soft drinks.

> Have you ever felt dizzy after a meal or when you've stood up suddenly? These sudden drops in blood pressure are called postprandial hypotension and postural hypotension. Drinking something caffeinated can counteract these episodes of low blood pressure by triggering a small, healthy rise in your blood pressure.

Calcium

milk • cheese • yogurt • cereal • spinach • legumes • oysters • sardines

Smile if you love calcium. Your teeth certainly do. Calcium also gives your bones — and your brain — plenty to smile about.

The most abundant mineral in your body, calcium is essential for strong bones and teeth. In fact, 99 percent of the calcium in your body is found in those areas.

But the other 1 percent does some pretty important things, too. Calcium helps regulate blood pressure and is needed for muscle contraction, including your heartbeat. It also plays a role in blood clotting, nerve transmission, and the secretion of hormones, digestive enzymes, and neurotransmitters.

An adult's daily recommended intake for calcium is 1,000 mg from ages 19-50 and 1,200 mg from age 51 and up. You can get plenty of calcium from your diet. Milk, cheese, and other dairy products are good sources, while legumes, greens, some breakfast cereals, sardines, and tofu also provide calcium. A variety of calcium supplements is also available.

Calcium gets most of its attention for protecting against osteoporosis, or brittle bone disease. But that's not the only reason to fit more calcium into your diet. Find out how the mineral that strengthens your bones and teeth also strengthens your mind.

1 cup Total Raisin Bran cereal	1,000 mg*
1 cup ricotta cheese	669 mg
8 oz. low-fat yogurt	415 mg
1 cup fat-free or skim milk	299 mg
1 cup cooked spinach	245 mg
1 oz. Swiss cheese	224 mg

* milligrams

4 ways calcium keeps you sharp

Boosts brain function. Studies suggest calcium plays a role in how your brain works. In a study of older, rural Chinese people, those with higher blood levels of calcium fared better on tests of mental function, including memory and learning.

A French study found that high concentrations of calcium in drinking water protected against mental impairment in older men and women. Similarly, another study of older people in rural China noted that mental function increased with the calcium level of drinking water — but only until a certain point. Then it decreased as the calcium level increased.

On the other hand, Japanese researchers found that older women with Alzheimer's had significantly lower blood levels of calcium than women without dementia.

Researchers aren't sure exactly how calcium affects the brain. One possible explanation is that increased blood calcium levels enhance dopamine synthesis, and increased dopamine levels regulate various brain functions.

In animal tests, exercise boosts blood calcium levels. So in addition to getting more calcium into your diet, maybe you should get moving to reap the brain benefits of this important mineral.

> Adding calcium to your diet is especially important if you're prone to kidney stones. That's because calcium binds with oxalate in your gut, preventing its absorption in your body. A diet low in calcium and high in oxalate is a recipe for disaster. If you have kidney stones, avoid foods high in oxalate, including spinach, rhubarb, beets, black tea, chocolate, nuts, wheat bran, and legumes.

Helps your heart. What's good for your heart is also good for your brain — and calcium benefits your heart in several ways. If you're concerned about high blood pressure, you probably know cutting back on sodium while boosting potassium can help lower it.

Now you can add calcium to the mix. Calcium lowers blood pressure in both healthy people and those with high blood pressure. Getting more calcium into your diet even slows the rise of systolic blood pressure (the top number in a blood pressure reading) that comes with age.

But calcium's heart-healthy benefits don't stop there. A New Zealand study of older women found that calcium supplements boosted levels of high-density lipoprotein (HDL), or good cholesterol, by 7 percent. In another study, dieters who took calcium along with vitamin D lowered their low-density lipo-protein (LDL), or bad cholesterol, by 14 percent.

Not surprisingly, considering its positive effects on blood pressure and cholesterol, calcium also protects against stroke, or brain attack. A Japanese study found that a high intake of dietary calcium, especially from dairy products, reduced the risk of stroke in middle-age men and women.

A University of California, Los Angeles study suggested that calcium can lessen the severity of strokes and make recovery go more smoothly. People who had high blood levels of calcium had strokes one-third as severe as those with relatively low levels. They also were much less likely to function poorly by the time they left the hospital.

Watches your weight. Slimming down may help you smarten up. Obesity has been linked to Alzheimer's disease and other forms of dementia. Of course, being overweight also puts you at greater risk for heart disease and diabetes — conditions that also affect your brain. Several studies suggest that calcium helps you lose weight or keep your weight under control.

One study found that calcium supplements may help control women's weight in middle age, while another suggested that the equivalent of two more servings of dairy a day could slash the risk of being over-weight by up to 70 percent. But it may not be that simple.

To get the weight-loss benefit of calcium, you still need to cut calories. That's the basis of any effective weight-loss plan. And the people who benefit the most from calcium are overweight people whose calcium intake was low to begin with. If you're not getting enough calcium, boosting your dairy intake while cutting calories could help you shed some pounds and reduce body fat.

Scientists aren't exactly sure why calcium aids weight loss. It may help control your appetite, block fat absorption, or suppress the hormone calcitrol, which can trigger fat buildup. It's likely several factors are involved.

Defends against diabetes. When you have diabetes, your glucose and insulin levels are out of whack. This can wreak havoc with your brain. High blood sugar levels impair your thinking and memory, and a lack of insulin has been linked to Alzheimer's disease. People with diabetes are more likely to have heart disease, which can cut off blood flow to your brain. They are also more likely to suffer from depression.

A recent study of Chinese women found that calcium and low-fat milk both protected against type 2 diabetes. This could be because of calcium's beneficial effect on body weight. Calcium is also essential for insulin-related processes in skeletal muscle and fat tissue. Milk, rich in calcium and vitamin D, may affect insulin sensitivity.

Boost your intake wisely

You should be getting 1,200 milligrams (mg) of calcium each day if you are over age 50. But where you get your calcium could make a difference.

A recent Washington University study found that women who got calcium primarily from their diet or from both food and supplements had healthier bones than those who got their calcium primarily from supplements. One theory is that calcium from food is more readily absorbed than calcium from supplements.

Should you opt to take calcium supplements, choose calcium carbonate or calcium citrate. Calcium carbonate is the most common and cheapest option. Take it with meals for better absorption. Go with calcium citrate if you have a condition called achlorhydria, a lack of stomach acid, or if you have inflammatory bowel disease or absorption disorders. You can take calcium citrate with or without food. To boost absorption of calcium supplements, do not take more than 500 mg at one time.

Thirsty for more calcium? You don't have to drink milk. High-calcium mineral waters are another good option. So are fortified beverages, like orange juice and rice milk. Just make sure to shake these beverages first. Otherwise, the added calcium can settle on the bottom of the container.

Drawbacks of too much calcium

Calcium has many health benefits, but you can get too much of a good thing. Experts have set the tolerable upper limit at 2,500 milligrams (mg) a day.

Too much calcium can lead to headache, irritability, calcium deposits in soft tissue, and even kidney failure. It also inhibits the absorption of other key minerals, like iron, magnesium, phosphorus, and zinc. If you take calcium supplements, you may also experience constipation, bloating, and gas.

Calcium interacts with some antibiotics, including tetracycline and ciprofloxacin, so you have trouble absorbing both the mineral and the drug. Skip calcium supplements until you finish your course of antibiotics.

Cottage cheese is a healthy, low-fat, protein-rich snack. But it may not provide as much calcium as you'd expect. Cottage cheese retains only 25 to 50 percent of the calcium of the milk it's made from. One cup of low-fat cottage cheese gives you 138 milligrams of calcium, less than half as much as you'd get from a cup of milk.

One recent New Zealand study even suggested that older women taking calcium supplements were more likely to suffer a heart attack or stroke. But other studies have found no such link.

Recent studies have also shown that high calcium intake does not prevent fractures. One reason could be that the women in the study were already getting enough calcium, and the extra calcium didn't do any good. In fact, if it blocked the absorption of phosphorus, it could have a negative effect on bone strength. Boosting your calcium may not help if your vitamin D levels are low, since you need vitamin D to absorb calcium.

Chinese emperors, Roman Emperor Nero, and adventurer Marco Polo all had their hands in the invention of ice cream. They used snow and honey to make a sweet, frozen concoction. Fortunately, you can satisfy your sweet tooth and get a bowlful of calcium with much less effort. Try this simple solution.

Do-it-yourself ice cream

1/2 cup milk

1/2 cup heavy cream

3 tsp. sugar or sugar substitute (add more if you like)

1/2 tsp. vanilla extract

Combine milk, heavy cream, and sweetener. Add vanilla extract.

Mix the ingredients in a sandwich-size zip-lock bag and seal the bag tightly. Place the small bag inside a gallon-size zip-lock bag filled just over half way with ice. Cover the ice with salt (kosher or ice cream salt is best, but table salt will do). Use enough salt to cover well. Close the bag tightly.

Gently shake the bag with the salt, ice, and little bag about 8 minutes until the ice cream solidifies. Don't knead the bag or the little bag could open.

Makes 2 servings

Complex carbohydrates

starchy vegetables • whole-grain rice • whole-grain breads • whole-grain cereals • beans • lentils • peas

Every body needs some carbohydrates. They are your most basic source of energy, fueling your brain and nervous system, in particular. But what about this anti-carb movement that's produced numerous diet books and eating plans? If you're more nutrition savvy than most, you know that not all carbohydrates are created equal. Lumping all of them into the bad-for-you category means you're missing out on foods teeming with essential vitamins, minerals, and fiber. Here's what you need to know.

Natural sugars like fructose, lactose, and maltose are considered simple carbs because of their chemical structure and the fact they break down quickly in your body. You'll find them in fruit, dairy, and some vegetables. Sounds healthy enough, but mostly because these foods contain other nutrients. Simple carbs are also the main ingredient in candy, soda, syrup, and table sugar or sucrose. They provide energy from calories but not much else. These are the carbohydrates you need to stay away from.

1 complex carbohydrate serving equals:
1 cup raw vegetables
1/2 cup cooked vegetables
1 baked potato or sweet potato
1 slice whole-wheat bread
2/3 cup whole-grain, ready-to-eat cereal
1/2 cup cooked brown rice
1/2 cup whole-wheat pasta
1/2 cup cooked beans, lentils, or peas

The carbs you should embrace are called complex. Foods containing them used to be known as starches, but healthy complex carbs are light-years away from the starches of your youth — soft white bread or polished white rice, for example. What you want are unrefined natural foods that break down slowly in your digestive system, release their sugars gradually, add bulk to your diet, and provide your body with a treasure trove of vitamins and minerals. Potatoes and other

Get about half your total calories from carbohydrates, preferably complex carbohydrates and natural sugars.

vegetables, whole grains, and peas and beans are great examples.

Experts may recommend a certain number of carbohydrate grams a healthy person should get every day, but beware. The source of these carb grams is almost more important than the amount.

Say you want to follow the Recommended Dietary Allowance of 130 grams (g) of carbohydrates a day. You can get about 50 g of carbs from either a half-cup of raisins or a half-cup of semi-sweet chocolate candies. And a cup of beans has the same amount of carbs as a slice of lemon meringue pie.

See the problem? These numbers show no distinction between simple and complex carbs. Use common sense and consider the amount of fiber in a food. That can be a better gauge of whether or not you could consider it a healthy complex carbohydrate.

5 ways complex carbohydrates keep you sharp

Blasts away a bad mood. Carbohydrates are feel-good foods. They naturally stimulate your body to produce serotonin, a brain chemical that affects, among other things, your mood. That explains why you get a little mental lift after you eat a carbohydrate-rich snack, like potato chips or pastries. And why, when you're stressed, you crave something sweet or starchy.

This can be a vicious cycle if you're feeling down because you're overweight. Simple carbs like these can pick you up, but they also contain a lot of empty calories. Choose complex carbs instead, like whole grains, and you've just tapped into a smart, healthy way to battle the blues.

Balances your blood sugar. If you suffer from diabetes, your goal is to keep a steady, controlled level of sugar in your blood. You don't want sudden spikes or crashing lows. All carbs contain sugars, but simple carbohydrates are broken down into these sugars faster. That means you get a sudden rush of sugar and energy followed by a hunger slump. Complex carbs are made up of larger molecules and break down into their component parts more slowly, releasing sugar and energy over a longer period of time.

Peps up your life. Carbohydrates keep you full of vim and vigor in two ways.

- More get-up-and-go. They are your body's main source of fuel. Enzymes break the carbs down into glucose, also known as blood sugar, which your cells need to perform even the most basic of functions.

- Better sleep. Just as carbs are necessary to keep you moving, oddly enough, they can also help you rest. That's important for good daytime energy. Complex carbs cue your brain to pump out more serotonin. And one of serotonin's other jobs is to promote relaxation and good sleep.

Helps you recall it all. Need another reason to keep complex carbohydrates on the menu? Think for a minute what it means to your brain cells when their main source of energy, glucose, is cut off. Women in a Tufts University study completely eliminated carbs from their diet then took part in tests of their brainpower. They scored worse on memory tests than women who were following a low-calorie diet. As the first group gradually added carbs back into their diet, their memory scores improved.

Encourages healthy weight loss. You may lose some weight if you go on a no-carbohydrate diet, but health professionals are fairly convinced you won't keep it off. Certainly you're eliminating all those unhealthy sugars in simple carbs, but you're also missing out on the nutrients and fiber in complex carbs.

More than 4,000 Canadians participated in a study to test the theory behind those no-carb diets, and the results should have you cooking up some whole-wheat pasta. Those who ate the least carbohydrates were more likely to be overweight, while people eating up to 300 carbohydrate grams a day were more likely to be slim. This isn't a case of more is better, however. Those who ate more than 300 grams of carbs daily were also more likely to carry extra pounds.

A cup of black beans provides a whopping 15 grams of fiber. Mix them with tomatoes and spices and you have a tasty chili treat that will keep you warm and give you lasting energy.

Quick black bean chili

1 lb. ground beef chuck, turkey, or chicken
1 medium onion, diced
1 15-oz. can chili-ready tomatoes
1 15-oz. can beef broth
1 15-oz. can black beans
1 tsp. pepper
3 tbsp. ketchup
10 dashes Louisiana hot sauce, Tabasco, or small can of peppers
Salt to taste

In a large, deep skillet or wok, brown the meat and onions, adding the salt, pepper, and hot sauce.

Add the beans, tomatoes, and broth and simmer on low for about 45 minutes, stirring occasionally.

Makes 4 servings

Nutrition labels cut the carb confusion

There's a simple way to tell if a food contains healthy, complex carbohydrates or the not-so-good, simple variety. Look at its nutrition label. You'll see an entry for Total Carbohydrate. A high number here may be good news.

To be sure, glance just below to the Dietary Fiber and Sugars entries. Which line has the bigger number? If you've got more fiber than sugar, chances are this food is a healthy choice for complex carbohydrates. If the sugar number is high, you're looking at a lot of unhealthy, simple carbohydrate grams. Compare the two carbohydrate entries in the nutrition labels below.

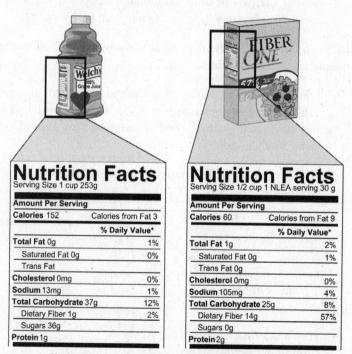

Nutrition Facts
Serving Size 1 cup 253g

Amount Per Serving

Calories 152	Calories from Fat 3
	% Daily Value*
Total Fat 0g	1%
Saturated Fat 0g	0%
Trans Fat	
Cholesterol 0mg	0%
Sodium 13mg	1%
Total Carbohydrate 37g	12%
Dietary Fiber 1g	2%
Sugars 36g	
Protein 1g	

Nutrition Facts
Serving Size 1/2 cup 1 NLEA serving 30 g

Amount Per Serving

Calories 60	Calories from Fat 9
	% Daily Value*
Total Fat 1g	2%
Saturated Fat 0g	1%
Trans Fat 0g	
Cholesterol 0mg	0%
Sodium 105mg	4%
Total Carbohydrate 25g	8%
Dietary Fiber 14g	57%
Sugars 0g	
Protein 2g	

Nutritional data and images courtesy of www.NutritionData.com

Scientists shed light on sugar myths

Stop panicking over high-fructose corn syrup (HFCS). There are other issues you should panic about — things like:

- the total amount of sugars you're getting. Older women who aren't very active should get only about three teaspoons of added sugar a day. Most people get an average of 22.

- how prevalent sugars are in processed foods. Soft drinks are the major source of added sugars for Americans, with one can containing about eight teaspoons of sugar.

- the epidemic of obesity in the United States. An extra 50 calories a day — or three additional teaspoons of sugar — could mean up to a 5-pound weight gain in a year.

HFCS is no better or worse than most other sweeteners. Here are some points to keep in mind.

- HFCS is about 55 percent fructose and 45 percent glucose. Table sugar, also known as sucrose, is 50 percent fructose and 50 percent glucose. The two sweeteners are almost identical chemically.

- HFCS, table sugar, and honey all are digested and metabolized similarly.

- All sugars — HFCS, sucrose, fructose, and glucose — have the same number of calories, four in 1 gram or about 16 calories per teaspoon.

- HFCS is a different animal from pure fructose. Many alarming studies on pure

> Potatoes are a good source of complex carbohydrates. That's a good thing because Americans eat a lot of them — about 130 pounds per person every year. Just choose healthy dishes and stay away from chips and fries.

fructose used enormous amounts in rats, sometimes 60 percent of their daily energy. That's at least four times the amount in a normal human diet.

- Whether you're talking about sugar or HFCS, too much is unhealthy.

Curcumin

battles Alzheimer's disease • fights cancer • reduces inflammation • soothes arthritis • heals heartburn • combats diabetes • guards your heart • controls weight

Music and medicine have changed a lot over the years — and not always for the better. Just as you may prefer listening to the songs of yesteryear over the latest pop hits, you may prefer time-tested, ancient remedies to modern drugs. Tune in to turmeric, a spice popular in India and southern Asia, for a good example.

Turmeric, an important ingredient in curry powder, has been used for flavor and food coloring for thousands of years, dating back to 600 B.C. It has even been used in traditional Indian medicine to treat stomach disorders, arthritis pain, and low energy. But this ancient spice has very modern health benefits, as well.

Curcumin, a compound found in turmeric, is the key. It gives dishes made with turmeric and curry powder their distinctive yellow color, but it also provides so much more. The strong antioxidant and anti-inflammatory powers of curcumin make it a dynamo against a wide range of conditions.

Studies suggest curcumin helps fight several types of cancer, arthritis, Crohn's disease, diabetes and its complications, heart problems, high cholesterol, obesity, and heartburn.

Curcumin also protects your brain. Find out how this mighty compound can spice up your defense against Alzheimer's disease and other threats.

4 ways curcumin keeps you sharp

Attacks Alzheimer's disease. India has the lowest rate of Alzheimer's in the world. It could be because people there use so much of one spice — turmeric. Of course, genetics and other lifestyle factors could also make a difference, but there is some scientific support for this spicy link.

Lab studies show that curcumin stops brain plaques from forming and even breaks them down. In a small University of California, Los Angeles study, curcumin boosted the effectiveness of macrophages, your immune system's garbage men that travel through your brain and body cleaning up waste products. After being treated with curcumin, the macrophages of people with Alzheimer's disease did a better job of whisking away beta-amyloid, the protein deposits that form plaques.

Feel a cold coming on? Reach for the turmeric. To treat a sore throat, people in India add some turmeric to warm milk. That's because curcumin can help fight infections. In fact, topical turmeric even helps with wound healing.

Another study found that curcumin worked well with vitamin D3 to prevent the buildup of beta-amyloid in people with Alzheimer's disease, although synthetic versions of curcumin worked better than the natural form. Other studies show that curcumin reduces oxidative stress and inhibits inflammatory proteins that can harm your brain.

The combination of curcumin's antioxidant, anti-inflammatory, and immune-boosting powers makes it an ideal weapon against Alzheimer's disease.

A National University of Singapore study provides more evidence for the link. In the study, which included more than 1,000 Asian people between ages 60 and 93, those who ate curry occasionally or often performed better on mental tests than those who ate curry rarely or never.

The good news is a little curry goes a long way. For the study, "often" simply meant more than once a month and "occasionally" meant at least once in six months but less than once a month.

Defends against diabetes. High blood sugar can put your brain at high risk. Fortunately, curcumin may help protect against diabetes. In a Korean study, curcumin lowered blood sugar and acted as a powerful antioxidant in diabetic mice. It also lowered cholesterol and triglycerides.

An extract of turmeric called turmeric oleoresin, which contains both curcumin and turmeric essential oil, fights high blood sugar and abdominal fat in mice. Curcumin on its own also reduces high blood sugar.

In a promising new diabetes treatment, an Australian researcher developed an injection of curcumin coated in absorbable fat. The curcumin targets liver cells to prevent their inflammation. This inflammation occurs with obesity and often leads to diabetes. While the injection works in mice, it has not yet been tested on humans.

Diabetes often comes with complications, and curcumin can help with those, too. In a study of rats, turmeric and curcumin delayed the progression and maturation of cataracts caused by high blood sugar. Their antioxidant powers get the credit.

Oxidative stress and inflammation contribute to the development of diabetic retinopathy, a major cause of blindness. Curcumin reduces oxidative stress and inflammation in diabetic rats, which suggests that it could protect against diabetic retinopathy.

In an Indian study, the combination of insulin and curcumin relieved pain in mice with diabetic neuropathy, or nerve damage caused by high blood sugar.

Helps your heart. If you love your brain, take care of your heart. Many heart-related problems, including high blood pressure and high cholesterol, can become brain-related problems. Curcumin has a few heart-healthy properties.

An enlarged heart means an enlarged risk for heart attack or heart failure. In a Canadian study, curcumin prevented and even reversed enlarged heart in mice. Japanese researchers have reported similar results in studies of rats.

Curcumin may also protect your arteries from fatty buildup. A recent French study found that mice fed a diet supplemented with curcumin showed a 26 percent reduction in fatty deposits compared to mice on a standard diet. In an Indian study, curcumin boosted good HDL cholesterol levels while lowering total cholesterol. High cholesterol raises your risk of Alzheimer's, and cholesterol may help beta-amyloid proteins clump together in plaques.

> Mix turmeric and black pepper to make a tasty rub for fish and chicken. As a bonus, this combination boosts your body's absorption of curcumin.

Overcomes obesity. Losing weight can keep you from losing your mind. Obesity increases your risk for diabetes and heart disease, as well as dementia.

A recent study found that curcumin helps lower body fat and weight gain. Mice fed a high-fat diet supplemented with curcumin reduced weight gain and body fat even though their food intake was the same as the other group on a high-fat diet. The curcumin-fed mice also had lower blood sugar, triglycerides, and cholesterol. Curcumin may work in part by stopping the growth of new blood vessels in fat tissue.

In a recent lab study, curcumin — along with resveratrol — reduced inflammation in fat tissue. This kind of chronic inflammation can lead to heart disease and diabetes.

The lowdown on spices, supplements, and sprays

Curcumin comes in a variety of forms, giving you a few ways to benefit from this powerful compound.

You don't have to venture beyond the spice aisle of your grocery store to find turmeric and curry powder. Adding more of these spices to your diet will boost your curcumin intake. Pure turmeric powder will give you the most curcumin, while the curcumin content of curry powder varies greatly.

The average Indian eats about 2 to 2.5 grams of turmeric a day — which means about 60 to 200 milligrams (mg) of curcumin. If your taste buds can't handle all that spice, you can always take turmeric or curcumin supplements.

When shopping for supplements, pay attention to product labels, which should indicate which part of the plant was used. Look for root or rhizome powder or extract. Also look for curcumin concentration. Typical dosages range from 450 mg of curcumin capsules to 3 grams of turmeric root daily, divided into several doses.

You can even find curcumin in the form of Curecumin nasal or oral sprays.

Curcumin cautions

While turmeric or curcumin supplements are generally considered safe, they do have some drawbacks. They may cause upset stomach, nausea, or diarrhea. You may also experience an allergic skin reaction, such as an itchy rash.

Do not take these supplements if you are also taking blood thinners or if you have gallstones or gallbladder disease. They may increase bleeding and cause your gallbladder to contract.

A recent Wake Forest study found that curcumin can affect iron metabolism, especially in people with borderline iron deficiency. If you have anemia, you may want to rethink taking curcumin supplements.

Remember, herbs and dietary supplements are not strictly regulated by the FDA, so you're not always sure what you're getting. As always, talk to your doctor before taking any supplements.

Depression

sadness • loss of interest • feelings of worthlessness
• fatigue • sleep problems

Everyone feels sad sometimes or occasionally has trouble getting out of bed in the morning. But if you have depression, you feel sad almost all the time and may not be able to get out of bed. Depression is a serious condition that can drastically affect your everyday life.

When you have depression, you can't just cheer up or "snap out of it." Your sad mood lingers, you lose interest in activities you previously enjoyed, and you feel worthless. You may also experience fatigue, sleep problems, changes in appetite and weight, indecisiveness, and thoughts of death or suicide.

Several factors can contribute to depression, including genetics, drug or alcohol abuse, medications, and other medical conditions. Changes in your brain play a major role. Specifically, imbalances in the neurotransmitters serotonin, norepinephrine, and dopamine affect your mood. These chemicals act as messengers within your brain, so an imbalance can send the wrong message. Chronic inflammation in the brain may also be to blame.

Depression doesn't just affect your mood. It also takes a toll on your body, raising your risk of heart disease and death and aggravating chronic conditions like diabetes, arthritis, back problems, and asthma. It may even be an early signal of Alzheimer's disease.

Older people are particularly at risk. That's because life changes, like retirement or the loss of a spouse, can trigger depression. Social isolation, chronic illnesses, and prescription drugs can also make you depressed.

The most common treatment for depression includes antidepressant medication and therapy. But you can also take some steps to brighten your mood.

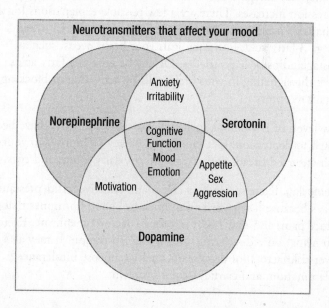

5 tactics to fight depression

Boost your mood with food. What you eat can affect how you feel. Change your diet, and you may change your mood for the better.

Japanese researchers found that men who ate the most carbohydrates were much less likely to show symptoms of depression than those who ate the least. A high intake of carbohydrates helps deliver the amino acid tryptophan to your brain, which stimulates the synthesis of serotonin. Choose complex carbohydrates, like whole grains and starchy vegetables, and healthy, simple carbohydates, like fruit and honey.

Citrus fruits and other brightly colored fruits and vegetables, rich in antioxidants like vitamin C and carotenoids, also help by protecting your brain from oxidative stress, which contributes to depression.

Omega-3 fatty acids, found in fish, also fight depression. As a population's omega-3 consumption decreases, its incidence of depression increases. There are a few possible explanations for this. Perhaps your brain converts eicosapentaenoic acid (EPA), an omega-3 fatty acid, into chemicals your brain needs, such as prostaglandins or leukotrienes. Or maybe omega-3 fatty acids affect the signaling in your brain cells by activating or blocking certain receptors.

Low levels of B vitamins such as folate or vitamin B12 have been linked to depression. Get more of these key vitamins into your diet with enriched breads and cereals, meats, dairy foods, and eggs.

Get moving. Exercise can be a cheap and effective antidepressant. That's because it releases endorphins, feel-good hormones that reduce pain, and may boost serotonin or norepinephrine. Exercise also helps you reduce stress, anger, and frustration. It may also lower risk factors for depression, such as glucose intolerance, inflammation, and cardiovascular problems.

You don't need to join a gym or buy special equipment. Just walking does the trick. Even everyday activities like housework — as long as they last at least 20 minutes and make you feel out of breath — can help.

One recent study found that the mood-lifting benefits of exercise last as long as 12 hours. Make sure to exercise regularly to maintain those benefits. Aim for at least 30 minutes a day, but every bit helps.

Be on the lookout for warning signs of suicide. Red flags include threatening or talking about suicide, feelings of hopelessness, rage or uncontrolled anger, feeling trapped, increased substance abuse, withdrawing from friends and family, acting reckless, and dramatic mood changes. For help, call the National Suicide Prevention Lifeline at 800-273-TALK.

Snooze to lose the blues. Insomnia may be a symptom or a cause of depression. Not getting enough sleep and poor sleep habits can make your depression worse and interfere with your treatment.

Improve your mood by improving the quality of your sleep. Helpful tips for better sleep include sticking to a regular sleep schedule; exercising regularly but not too close to bedtime; avoiding late-afternoon naps; keeping your bedroom dark, quiet, and cool; using your bed only for sleeping and sex; and avoiding caffeine and alcohol at night.

Focus on friendship. The Beatles put it well — you can get by with a little help from your friends. Social isolation can contribute to depression, but a strong support system can help you cope with life's ups and downs. Stay connected to friends and family or get involved with church groups or a local senior center.

You might even "catch" happiness from a friend or family member. A recent study found that being close to happy people increases your chances of becoming happy, too.

Sample some supplements. Try a safe, natural alternative to prescription drugs. Some supplements may help get you out of the doldrums — without unpleasant side effects.

Several clinical trials and reviews of studies have determined that St. John's wort works better than a placebo and just as well as standard antidepressants for mild to moderate depression. This herbal remedy may work by inhibiting the reuptake of serotonin, dopamine, and norepinephrine. This means that, rather than being reabsorbed and recycled by the cells that originally produced them, these chemicals remain in your brain to boost your mood.

> Savor simple pleasures. According to a Cleveland Clinic study, listening to music can ease depression symptoms by 25 percent. Gardening may also lift your spirits. A British study found that friendly bacteria commonly found in soil triggers your brain to produce serotonin.

S-adenosyl-methionine, better known as SAM-e, may also combat depression. SAM-e, a natural compound found in every cell of your body, has antioxidant and anti-inflammatory powers. It even helps in the production of neurotransmitters. In a recent 30-person study, Harvard researchers found that SAM-e helped some severely depressed people who did not respond to traditional medications.

Sidestep dangerous herb-drug interactions

St. John's wort may work as well as some prescription drugs, but it doesn't always work well with them. Beware of interactions. This herb can weaken the power of many medications, including cholesterol-lowering drugs, blood pressure drugs, and blood thinners.

If you take St. John's wort along with selective serotonin reuptake inhibitors (SSRIs), such as Prozac or Zoloft, it may trigger a dangerous condition called serotonin syndrome. You might become confused, hot, sweaty, and restless and experience headaches, stomachaches, muscle spasms, or seizures.

SSRIs, although considered the safest class of antidepressants, come with their own risks. Side effects include anxiety, nervousness, insomnia, drowsiness, nausea, and sexual problems. They may also increase your risk of stomach bleeding, especially when taken with nonsteroidal anti-inflammatory drugs like ibuprofen or aspirin. Older people taking SSRIs are more likely to fall, and SSRIs may weaken your bones, making you more prone to fractures.

A word of caution — never stop taking a drug your doctor prescribed without his approval.

SAD news you can use

You may have seasonal affective disorder, or SAD, if you're depressed in the late fall and winter. The diminished daylight hours can mess up your body's internal clock. Ask your doctor about light therapy, which involves sitting in front of a special lamp that uses multiple full-spectrum fluorescent lights.

The key is the bright artificial light, measured in units called lux. Typical therapy is 2,500 lux for two hours a day or 10,000 lux for 30 minutes a day. Notice how that compares to other common sources of light, including sunlight and home lighting.

Light Source	Lux
Sunlight at noon	100,000
Hazy day	50,000
SAD light therapy	10,000
SAD light therapy	2,500
Overcast day	2,000
Office	200-500
Living room	50-200
Average nursing home	50
Full moon	1

Diabetes

frequent urination • unusual thirst • infections
• blurred vision • fatigue • tingling
• numbness • slow-healing cuts

There's a power struggle going on in your body right now between glucose and insulin. Do you know who is winning? If you suffer from diabetes, your insulin may be down for the count.

Glucose is a sugar that provides the energy your cells need to function. Important stuff. You get some glucose from the foods you eat and some is produced by your liver. Insulin, on the other hand, is like the switchman for your body's energy train. It tells your liver how much glucose to produce and helps move the glucose from your bloodstream into your cells. When everything is working properly, your pancreas makes the right amount of insulin and your cells get the right amount of glucose. Everything is in sync in your body and you feel fine. If you have type 2 diabetes, however, the balance of power is upset.

Some say there are three stages to diabetes.

- First, you develop insulin resistance, which means insulin has trouble moving glucose into receptor cells where it can be used. Most people compensate for this by making more insulin to overcome this resistance.

- Over time, your pancreas simply can't keep up, and you don't produce enough insulin when you need it. The amount of glucose in your blood varies wildly depending on how much insulin you have and how well it is working.

- Eventually, all that excess glucose in your bloodstream destroys the insulin-producing cells in your pancreas, and you develop full-blown diabetes.

So what does that mean to your overall health? Fluctuations in the amount of glucose in your blood can wreak havoc on your entire body. Everything from your ears to your feet can be affected. But damage to your brain may be the scariest part of all.

When your blood glucose levels spike, you can immediately experience any number of side effects that impact your mental abilities — like dehydration and fatigue. If your levels drop, you may feel confused and uncoordinated. You might experience a headache, double vision, or slurred speech. These are short-term symptoms that usually go away when your blood sugar stabilizes. However, there are long-term complications of diabetes that also affect your brain and mental health. Every time your blood sugar swings high or low, there is minor damage to your body that can ultimately lead to serious problems.

High blood glucose levels can injure the inside of your artery walls, leading to plaque deposits and reduced blood flow. The bad news for you — impaired blood flow increases your risk of a stroke or heart attack. In fact, if you have diabetes, you're two to four times more likely to suffer from heart disease than someone without diabetes.

But can diabetes affect how well you think and remember? You bet. As your blood sugar levels rise, your ability to think quickly and multitask decline. There are several possible explanations for this. If glucose isn't getting into your brain cells, they don't have enough energy to function properly. And neurons that aren't working mean a brain that's not working. This kind of cognitive damage sets you up for a vicious cycle of decline.

Tag! You have diabetes. There's a new screening tool in town called TAG-IT (the Tool to Assess Likelihood of Fasting Glucose Impairment). It's easy and fast. And it could save your life. You answer six questions about yourself and your health, and you receive an overall risk score that lets a doctor know if you should be further screened for diabetes.

When your thinking is impaired, you may not take your diabetes medication properly, eat right, or remember to exercise. Your diabetes gets worse, which further impacts your mental abilities.

In addition, new research finds that both diabetes and Alzheimer's disease (AD) are affected by a lack of insulin. Men who didn't produce the right amount of insulin at age 50 were at a significantly greater risk of developing AD and other types of dementia later on.

And if you just don't feel well, you can blame that on diabetes, too. People with diabetes have more than a 50 percent higher risk of depression. Some experts say the stress of trying to manage diabetes is depressing, while others believe inflammation and hormones may be to blame. Oddly enough, it's also true that if you are depressed, you're more likely to develop diabetes. This can be partially explained by lifestyle factors. For example, depressed people are more likely to smoke, be less physically active, and eat more.

Diet and exercise may not be enough to control blood glucose levels for some people. If you can't meet your HbA1c goal or if you develop diabetes symptoms, your doctor will probably start you on oral medications and, possibly, insulin injections.

4 tactics to fight diabetes

Lose weight. It's the single most important thing you can change about your diabetes risk. Experts say being overweight is the major contributing factor to type 2 diabetes, and if you carry extra fat around your middle, you're even more likely to develop diabetes than someone who is heavier in the hips and thighs. If you're trying to gauge your risk, don't just go by the scale. Take a tape measure to your waist.

Take charge of your blood pressure. There is no ideal weight for everyone, but there is a specific goal you should set when it comes to your blood pressure. Keep it lower than 130/80 mm Hg and you could prevent or delay diabetes complications. You might even reduce the severity of complications that do occur.

Know your cholesterol levels. You've learned how important a healthy heart is to fighting diabetes. That's why taking steps to control your cholesterol is one of the best ways to maintain a strong ticker and flexible blood vessels. Get your bad low-density lipoprotein (LDL) cholesterol below 100 mg/dL. Below 70 is even better. Triglycerides should be less than 150 mg/dL, and you want your good high-density lipoprotein (HDL) level to be at least around 50 mg/dL.

Keep blood sugar stable. You can actually monitor how much glucose is in your blood with a hemoglobin A1c (HbA1c) test administered every three to six months. Controlling blood sugar is, of course, what diabetes is all about — no spikes, no lows. You want to maintain your HbA1c levels at or below 7 percent.

But there is controversy over how important blood sugar control is, compared to other factors like cholesterol and blood pressure. Many health professionals think drastic measures to lower or maintain a certain glucose level is not as vital to diabetes management as controlling cholesterol levels and blood pressure.

One example of this controversy is the eating plan based on a glycemic index (GI). The GI measures how a carbohydrate-containing food raises your blood glucose. Foods are ranked based on how they compare to white bread. A food with a high GI raises blood glucose more than a food with a medium or low GI. This method of choosing foods can be complicated. Not only do you need to refer to a specific list, but a GI for one food can vary based on how it is prepared.

The American Diabetes Association takes a simpler approach to nutrition. They suggest eating a variety of foods, including fruits, vegetables, whole grains, nonfat dairy products, beans, lean meats, and fish. Always choose foods rich in vitamins, minerals, and fiber instead of nutrient-poor, processed foods.

The bottom line — make sensible, healthy choices, eating foods that provide key nutrients over unhealthier ones.

Choose this	Instead of this
peanut butter	high-fat lunch meat
coffee	soda
sweet potato	french fries
cinnamon	sugar
garlic	salt
berries	cookies
whole-wheat bread	pastry
beans	red meat

One last thought. Any time you're physically active, you're using glucose. That means there's less to accumulate in your bloodstream. In addition, exercise builds muscle and muscle cells need large amounts of glucose. Just one more reason to get up and get moving.

Simple blood test can save your life

Millions of people are teetering on the edge of diabetes and don't know it. They have a condition called prediabetes — which means their fasting blood glucose level is between 100 and 125 mg/dL. These numbers are higher than normal, but not high enough for most doctors to raise the alarm. If this is you, and you don't change your lifestyle or take medication, you're likely to develop type 2 diabetes within 10 years.

It's easy to get your glucose levels tested. There are three different blood tests your doctor can perform — casual plasma glucose, fasting plasma glucose (FPG), or oral glucose tolerance test. If you are over age 45, get tested. If you're under age 45, overweight, and have any other risk factors for diabetes, ask your doctor about testing.

> Remember to have your blood pressure checked every time you visit your doctor. And have your cholesterol level checked yearly or more often if you aren't at your target numbers.

Falls

dizziness • dehydration • impaired vision • muscle weakness • pets

A fall used to mean scraped knees and cartoon Band-Aids. Now that you're older, it can mean broken bones and head trauma. In fact, almost a third of seniors who fall suffer serious injuries.

If you fall and hit your head, it does more than just shake you up. It sets the stage for a slump in brain skills and increases your risk of Alzheimer's disease (AD) and other forms of dementia. How severe your particular outcome is depends in part on whether or not you lose consciousness. Experts say your risk of AD is almost 10 times higher if you black out from a head injury. If you're out for more than five minutes, you're more likely to develop AD earlier in life.

There are several possible explanations for how a blow to the head can impair your thinking. It could cause brain cells to die or damage the blood brain barrier, which protects your brain from foreign substances in your blood and from hormones and neurotransmitters in the rest of your body. It also helps maintain a controlled environment for your brain.

Simply becoming smart about your fall risk is an advantage. Studies show prevention programs for seniors resulted in 11 percent fewer falls. Read on for your own fall-avoidance game plan.

7 tactics to fight falls

Examine your medicine cabinet. While it's true the medications you take are supposed to fix a problem, sometimes they cause more problems. That's the case with certain sleeping pills, antidepressants, heart drugs, and some over-the-counter remedies for allergies and colds. They can make you drowsy or dizzy — and that makes you more apt to stumble. You're especially at risk if:

- you're taking an SSRI (selective serotonin reuptake inhibitor) for depression. In fact, you're 50 percent more likely to fall than other seniors.

- you're more sensitive to adverse or side effects of drugs.

- you're taking more than four medications.

Ask your doctor if a pill could be making you unsteady on your feet, or check things out online. Go to *www.worstpills.org* and conduct an advanced search by "Drug-Induced Disease or Condition." Select "dizziness" or "falls," and you'll see a list of drugs that might be rocking your world.

If you think a drug you are taking is affecting your balance, talk with your doctor. Never stop taking a drug your doctor prescribed without his approval.

Get your eyes and ears checked. You'll feel more secure if you can see and hear clearly. Have you visited your eye doctor lately? Make sure your glasses are the right prescription and get checked for glaucoma and cataracts.

Along those same lines, any problem with your inner ear can leave you feeling disoriented, causing dizziness, vertigo, and balance problems. You could have a simple ear infection or be suffering from allergies or Meniere's disease. The older you get, the more likely you are to have something go wrong in the delicate workings of your inner ear. More than one-third of Americans over age 40 have inner ear problems, also known as vestibular dysfunction. And if that's you, you're 12 times more likely to suffer a fall.

> Don't walk and talk. Don't walk and eat. Don't walk and text. For that matter, just walk. Studies prove if you try to "dual task," or walk and do anything else at the same time, you're five times more likely to fall.

Stay steady with proper footwear. It's a bit surprising, but experts say you're about 10 times more likely to fall if you walk around barefoot. Athletic shoes are best to keep you stabilized, either the kind that lace or those with Velcro fasteners. They need to fit properly and have good arch support, which boosts your balance and reduces joint pain. But stay away from extra-thick or slick soles. If you just can't stand to wear shoes in the house, don't resort to stocking feet. That's even more treacherous. Find an indoor shoe with a nonslip sole.

Improve balance through exercise. You have two goals here — strengthen the muscles in your lower body and improve your flexibility and range of motion. By accomplishing these, you'll gain the tools you need to stay steady and balanced. You've got lots of options, too. Yoga and tai chi can improve your balance and strength. But really, anything that gets you up and moving will fight the loss of muscle tone so common as people age. Use elastic bands on your legs and ankles for greater resistance. If you're not active because you're afraid of falling, think about this — physical activity can help prevent falls.

Fall-proof your home. One-half to two-thirds of all falls occur in or around the home. Cut your risk by taking a few simple precautions.

- Keep rooms well-lit, but don't have electrical or extension cords trailing across the floor.

- Remove clutter from walkways and stairs.

- Get rid of loose throw rugs or tape them down.

- Amp up bathroom safety with grab bars, a raised toilet seat, and nonslip floor and bath mats.

- Install night lights.

- Check handrails for sturdiness.

- Train pets to walk calmly and not jump around your feet.

- Install cordless phones throughout your house so you don't have to hurry to catch a call.

Drink, drink, drink. A few glasses of water could mean the difference between clear-headedness and a life-altering fall. Every system in your body depends on water because it carries nutrients and oxygen to your cells. When you're dehydrated, water moves out of your cells into your bloodstream in an attempt to keep your blood volume and your blood pressure at a safe level. If dehydration continues, your cells shrivel up and no longer work properly.

Your brain cells are particularly at risk since your brain is about 70 percent water. Eventually, without enough water, your blood pressure falls, and you feel lightheaded, dizzy, and confused. If you stand up suddenly while dehydrated, your lowered blood pressure increases your chances of fainting and falling. If you're older, you get dehydrated more easily because you generally have more body fat, which contains less water than lean tissue. Also, your sense of thirst isn't as well-tuned as it used to be, so you may not feel thirsty.

A major study out of England found that seniors in a residential care facility who boosted their daily water intake reduced falls by 50 percent. Here are some important points to remember.

- Drink before you feel thirsty.

- Include water-rich fruits and vegetables in your diet, like berries, watermelon, grapes, peaches, tomatoes, and lettuce.

- Monitor your urine. Pale yellow is good. Dark amber means drink.

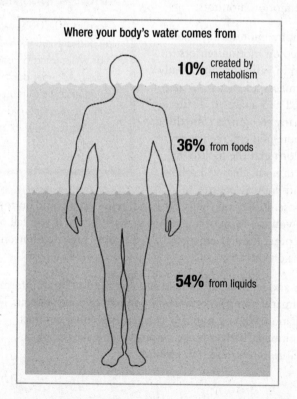

Where your body's water comes from

10% created by metabolism

36% from foods

54% from liquids

Decrease falls with vitamin D. This amazing vitamin is quite the multitasker. Not only does it help maintain healthy bones, it's important for muscle strength, as well. Without enough vitamin D, your muscles will hurt and feel weak, not good if you want to stand tall. Because older people aren't as efficient in processing vitamin D, you may be deficient and not know it. Talk to your doctor about supplements.

Get savvy to life-saving systems

There are two kinds of medical emergency alert systems you can use to "call" for help in case you fall — Personal Emergency Response Systems (PERS) and home motion monitors.

The home monitoring system is based on motion sensors placed in various rooms. Daily movements and activities are tracked and analyzed. If the company recognizes something as a potential emergency, say you don't exit the bathroom after an hour, they will follow up with a prearranged response. PERS, on the other hand, relies on a panic button usually in the form of a pendant or wrist band. If you fall or suffer some other kind of emergency, you simply press the button and help is on the way.

> Close to 50,000 seniors fall and are injured every year while using a cane or walker. Ask your doctor to spend extra time fitting you with your walking aid and teaching you how to use it safely.

Prices and services vary widely and you need to be an informed consumer if you plan on investing in one of these systems. There are installation fees and monthly charges. Ask about contract commitment, battery range, response time, repair policies, cancellation fees, and staff training.

Fatigue

physical or mental exhaustion • weakness
• lack of energy • poor sleep

It's an old joke that's not so funny — you're sick and tired of feeling sick and tired. Not surprisingly, there's nothing funny about persistent fatigue.

It's one of those "invisible" symptoms, like pain, that you can't prove to anyone — let alone your doctor. Face it, there's no medical test for fatigue. But there is a silver lining to your black cloud of exhaustion. Most times fatigue is a symptom of something else — not an illness all by itself. If you and your doctor can figure out what else is going on, you're on your way to recovery.

The first thing to check is your medicine cabinet. Are you taking a drug that leaves you feeling tired as a side effect? Antihistamines, blood pressure medicines, sleeping pills, steroids, and diuretics are prime suspects.

Talk to your pharmacist or doctor about a substitute if you think a drug you are taking is causing your fatigue. Don't stop taking the drug on your own.

You may be tempted to battle your fatigue with an age-old remedy — caffeine. But be careful if coffee becomes a necessary part of your routine. Relying on a stimulant for get-up-and-go can actually make your energy problem worse in the long run. Fix your fatigue with healthier tactics and drink caffeine occasionally because you want to — not because you need to.

It's also possible you're making certain lifestyle choices that are reducing your energy levels. Are you going to bed later than usual?

Are you feeling stressed, overworked, or bored? These are easy enough to fix if you examine your life and your schedule. Also consider these:

- poor nutrition, including dehydration

- lack of exercise

- overusing caffeine

That tired feeling could also stem from another illness. The list of potential offenders is long and varied. Everyday ailments, like allergies, chronic back pain, or an infection, can leave you drooping. Rare possibilities include stroke, multiple sclerosis, and Parkinson's disease. More common are these kinds of conditions that affect thousands of people:

- anemia

- hyperthyroidism or hypothyroidism

- heart disease

- diabetes

- kidney disease or liver disease

> Call your doctor right away if you feel unusually tired and have other disturbing symptoms like confusion, dizziness, blurred vision, recent weight gain, or little to no urine.

These underlying causes of fatigue affect your body's ability to function properly — all the way down to the cellular level in your blood and your brain. Because they affect your balance of nutrients, oxygen, and hormones, it's harder for you to concentrate, make decisions, solve problems, organize, multi-task, and process information.

Call your doctor if you have fatigue that lasts longer than two weeks. He'll probably recommend a thorough exam and some medical tests. If you're suffering from simple fatigue, here's how you can handle it on your own.

4 tactics to fight fatigue

Round out your menu. Fill up your body's gas tank with the right kind of fuel and you'll find it easier to get yourself in gear. Never skip breakfast and eat portion-controlled, healthy, well-balanced meals every three to four hours. Some health experts recommend taking a daily multivitamin. Want to talk specifics? Here's how different kinds of foods and nutrients keep your engine running.

- Carbohydrates supply glucose, an important energy source for almost everything going on inside your body.

- Protein provides about 10 percent of the total fuel you use whether you're at work or rest.

- Fiber regulates your digestion, giving you a steady release of energy.

- Fats are calorie-dense, with 1 gram of fat equaling nine calories. Unsaturated fats, like monounsaturated and poly-unsaturated, are healthy fats — as long as you eat them in moderation. Stored fat is your largest reserve of energy, providing the oomph you need for long, slow, low-intensity workouts, like cycling and walking.

- Iron gives oxygen a ride on its trip through your blood-stream. If your cells don't get enough oxygen, they can't produce energy.

Drink up. Water carries nutrients and oxygen to cells throughout your body. If you get dehydrated, even just a little, you'll feel tired and drained of energy. Participants in the Anglian Water study who tried to drink an extra two to eight glasses of water a day reported having more vim and vigor. Your best bet is to sip water all day long, but remember — you can get a lot of the fluids you need from foods like soup, juice, herbal tea, nonfat milk, fruits, and vegetables.

Get moving. When you're feeling sluggish, doing something active may be the last thing on your to-do list — but it should be the first. A new study out of the University of Georgia saw people increase their energy levels by 20 percent when they participated in regular, low-intensity exercise. Interestingly enough, the benefits don't stem so much from muscle or aerobic fitness, but from the way exercise acts on your central nervous system.

Rest well. Now that's what you really feel like doing — going to bed. But don't get too excited. You can't really fight fatigue by sleeping all the time. As long as your body isn't trying to fight some kind of illness or infection, you don't necessarily need more sleep. You just need an adequate amount of regular, restorative sleep. Nap if you need to, but go to bed on time and get up at the same time every morning. And do what you can to improve the quality of your sleep.

Fatigue and depression often go hand-in-hand, so much so that it's sometimes difficult to determine which one is causing the other. Feeling tired and listless all the time is enough to depress anyone. On the other hand, fatigue is a common side effect of depression, and many antidepressants can cause or worsen fatigue. Try to get an accurate diagnosis of your problem and discuss with your doctor the pros and cons of any medications.

Wise up to chronic fatigue's health risk

Unexplained fatigue that lasts more than six months and doesn't respond to rest or other traditional treatments is often called chronic fatigue syndrome (CFS). It's less common if you're under age 29 or over age 60, and women are more likely to experience CFS than men. Along with fatigue, you may experience memory or thinking problems, muscle or joint pain, sore throat, headaches, gastrointestinal problems, and depression.

It's a difficult diagnosis to make because it often occurs with other diseases. That's why most doctors will try to eliminate all other causes of your fatigue first. This is a complex, potentially serious condition, so if you feel you may be suffering from CFS, take it seriously and see your doctor.

Flavonoids

fruits • vegetables • legumes • tea • red wine
• chocolate • whole grains • herbs

Bite into a juicy fruit or a crisp vegetable, and you'll get more than you bargained for. Besides their valuable vitamins and minerals, fruits and vegetables also provide a host of beneficial substances called phytochemicals.

Phytochemicals, or plant chemicals, protect plants from weather, pests, and other dangers. But they may also protect you and your brain. Although they are not considered essential nutrients like vitamins, minerals, fat, protein, and carbohydrates, these substances still play an important role in your health. To highlight their importance — and to make them sound more appetizing — they are often called phytonutrients rather than phytochemicals.

There are thousands of phytonutrients, and many of them are classified as flavonoids. Like phytochemicals, flavonoids can be organized into several subclasses.

In general, flavonoids have antioxidant powers. They neutralize harmful free radicals and prevent metals, like iron, from creating them in the first place. They also affect cell signaling pathways to fight inflammation and control cell growth. Studies suggest they fight heart disease, cancer, and brain disorders.

Three specific types of flavonoids merit special attention.

- Anthocyanins. These pigments, which give foods their blue, red, or purple colors, give you plenty of health benefits. Found in berries, grapes, and red wine, anthocyanins have high antioxidant activity. They also thwart bad LDL cholesterol, prevent blood clotting, and guard against cancer.

- Catechins. The richest sources of catechins are tea and chocolate, but these flavonoids can also be found in grapes, berries, and apples. Epicatechins, which belong to the same subclass of flavonoids as catechins, also appear in these foods.

- Quercetin. One of the most abundant flavonoids, quercetin can be found in yellow onions, scallions, kale, broccoli, apples, berries, and teas.

While you can find these and other flavonoids in supplement form, your best bet may be to get them from colorful whole foods. That way, you get the full package. After all, whole foods are greater than the sum of their parts.

Read on to find out how each of these flavonoids — and the amazing fruits, vegetables, and other foods that contain them — can boost your brain and your health. You won't believe what's at the top of the list.

3 ways anthocyanins keep you sharp

Improve memory. Recent studies revealed some juicy news about anthocyanin-rich beverages.

One small study found that blueberry juice gives your memory a boost. In the 12-week study, nine older people with early memory decline drank the equivalent of about 2 1/2 cups of wild blueberry juice a day. Not only did their ability to learn and recall information improve, they also experienced fewer symptoms of depression and lowered their blood sugar levels.

The antioxidant and anti-inflammatory effects of the anthocyanins in blueberries may help protect your brain from decline. Anthocyanins may also increase brain signaling in areas of the brain related to memory.

Anthocyanin-rich foods	
1/2 cup elderberries	551 mg*
1/2 cup blueberries	121.36 mg
1 cup cranberries	91.88 mg
1 cup chopped red cabbage	65 mg
1/2 cup blackberries	64.8 mg
10 sweet cherries	64 mg
10 raspberries	61.56 mg
10 red grapes	22 mg

* milligrams

The same University of Cincinnati researchers also found positive results for Concord grape juice, another good source of anthocyanins.

Reverse brain aging. Every year, your birthday cake sports another candle, proving you can't stop the march of time. But you can go back in time for inspiration — and protection. Just eat more like our ancestors, who foraged for nuts and berries. Discover the nut and berry diet that could reverse brain aging.

Animal studies highlight the power of berries, which are great sources of anthocyanins. Blueberry extracts reduce oxidative stress and inflammation, which contribute to mental decline and dementia. They also reverse brain aging in older rats. In one study, blueberry and strawberry extracts counteracted the effects of radiation, which speeds up the aging process. Irradiated rats given blueberry or strawberry extracts navigated maze tests as well as rats that hadn't been radiated.

Recently, a study in England found that blueberries reverse age-related memory deficits in rats. Rats whose diets were supplemented with blueberry improved on spatial working memory tasks, which helped the rats find food at the end of the maze.

The credit goes to anthocyanins, which can cross the blood-brain barrier. Once there, they may enhance brain cell connections, improve communication between cells, and stimulate brain cell regeneration. Researchers speculate a link between anthocyanins and the activation of signaling proteins through a specific pathway in the hippocampus, the brain region that controls learning and memory.

Make room for a daily cup of blueberries, and you may reap the same benefits.

Include a handful of walnuts in your diet, and you'll protect your brain even more. Thanks to phytochemicals, including flavonoids, walnut extract stops beta-amyloid plaques from

Keep your eyes peeled for purple produce. These colorful versions of familiar foods provide an extra boost of healthy flavonoids. For example, Hawaiian purple sweet potatoes have 150 percent more anthocyanins than blueberries.

By activating snapdragon genes in tomato plants, scientists have created purple tomatoes rich in anthocyanins. Cancer-susceptible mice who ate the purple tomatoes lived significantly longer than those fed normal red tomatoes. You can also find purple cauliflower, which gets its color from anthocyanins.

forming and dissolves those already formed. These plaques represent a key feature of Alzheimer's disease.

According to a study of rats, walnuts may also improve balance, coordination, and memory. In the study, rats ate the human equivalent of an ounce of walnuts, or about seven to nine walnuts each day.

Conquer cholesterol. High cholesterol doesn't just put your heart in peril. It also endangers your brain, boosting your risk of dementia. Fortunately, anthocyanins can help save your heart and your brain.

Even better, anthocyanins are found in common foods that whisk artery-clogging cholesterol right out of your body. Chances are they're in your kitchen this very minute.

A Chinese study found that anthocyanins raise good HDL cholesterol by 13.7 percent while lowering bad LDL cholesterol by a nearly identical 13.6 percent. Since every 1 percent increase in HDL cholesterol and decrease in LDL cholesterol corresponds to a 1 percent reduction in heart disease risk, that means you can slash your risk of heart disease by 27.3 percent.

In the study, 120 people with high cholesterol between the ages of 40 and 65 took 160 milligrams of anthocyanins twice daily for 12 weeks. The anthocyanins used in the capsule — a mix of 17 different natural anthocyanins — came from bilberry and black currant.

Researchers speculate that anthocyanins may work by inhibiting cholesteryl ester transfer protein (CETP), which normally swaps cholesteryl ester from HDL with a harmful triglyceride molecule. Drugs called CETP inhibitors boost HDL and lower LDL, but they also raise blood pressure — while anthocyanins do not.

On the contrary, they may even help lower blood pressure. In a Finnish study, people who ate a variety of berries for two months lowered their systolic blood pressure — the top number in a blood pressure reading — and boosted their HDL cholesterol. On average, their HDL rose 5.2 percent and their systolic blood pressure dropped 1.5 points. But for people with high blood pressure, the drop was much more significant.

Berries eaten in the study included bilberries, lingonberries, black currants, strawberries, chokeberries, and raspberries. All rich in flavonoids, including anthocyanins, these berries were consumed whole, pureed, or in juice form.

Eating fruits and berries may also protect your blood vessels, according to a Norwegian study which measured the intima-media thickness (IMT) of the carotid artery, an indication of athero-sclerosis. Older men at risk for heart disease who ate the most fruits and berries had a 5.5 percent lower IMT compared to those who ate the least. Just one sweet fruit a day may help strengthen your blood vessels and raise your HDL cholesterol.

3 ways catechins keep you sharp

Boost your brain power. What is the best time of day to protect your brain? Tea time! A cup of tea can boost your brain power, but make sure you drink the right kind.

That means green tea, which contains more flavonoids — including catechins — than black or oolong teas. Green tea helps your brain in several ways.

One flavonoid in green tea called epigallocatechin-3-gallate (EGCG) reduced the formation of beta-amyloid proteins in the brains of mice with Alzheimer's disease. The buildup of beta-amyloid plaque likely contributes to the nerve damage and memory loss that comes with Alzheimer's disease. Other recent studies suggest green tea flavonoids may protect against Alzheimer's disease and Parkinson's disease, but more research is needed.

In a Japanese study, green tea catechins mixed with water improved learning ability and memory in rats. Researchers credit the antioxidant activity of catechins. By preventing oxidative stress, catechins help prevent mental decline.

Here's another way catechins give your brain a wake-up call. Sleep apnea robs you of a good night's rest. The disorder also drains your brain as you sleep, leaving your memory and learning ability impaired. In a recent University of Louisville study of rats, green tea catechins helped prevent these negative effects. For two weeks, rats were periodically deprived of oxygen during the night to simulate sleep apnea. Those whose water contained green tea catechins did much better on maze tests than those who drank plain water. They also

Catechin-rich foods	
1 cup green tea	300.11 mg*
1 cup oolong tea	117.74 mg
1 cup blueberries	76.53 mg
1 cup black tea	66.03 mg
1 cup blackberries	61.2 mg
1 oz. dark chocolate	14.98 mg
1 cup apple juice	14.78 mg
1 medium apple	13.81 mg
3 heaping teaspoons cocoa mix	7.34 mg

* milligrams

showed fewer signs of oxidative stress and inflammation. Sleep apnea can harm your brain — but green tea is the simple drink that may stop it.

Help your heart. Throw a tea party, and your heart will celebrate. That's because the catechins in tea protect your heart as well as your brain. And a healthy heart goes a long way toward keeping your brain healthy, too.

Drinking tea has been linked to lower rates of heart disease. Studies also suggest it may lower blood pressure, cholesterol, and triglycerides. Besides its well-known antioxidant and anti-inflammatory powers, tea also prevents blood clots and reduces cholesterol absorption.

A recent University of California, Los Angeles analysis determined that drinking three or more cups of green or black tea a day can lower your risk of stroke by 21 percent. While the mechanism remains unclear, the catechins in tea could be the key to tea's stroke-fighting ability.

Those same three daily cups of green tea can also reduce your risk of heart attack by an estimated 11 percent, according to another analysis of seven previous studies.

Trim the fat. Keeping off extra pounds can give your brain an extra boost. Obesity not only increases your risk of heart disease, stroke, and diabetes, it also ups your chances of developing dementia. Luckily, a cup of green tea may be a natural weight-loss aid.

A Dutch review of 11 studies found that green tea catechins significantly decreased body weight and successfully maintained body weight after weight loss. In a 12-week Japanese study, green tea extract containing 690 milligrams of catechins reduced body fat. People in the green tea group also had significantly lower body weight and slimmer waists than those in the control group.

By controlling your weight, you help reduce your risk of developing type 2 diabetes. But green tea may help in other ways, too. Some studies show that green tea flavonoids have positive effects on insulin activity. Even if you already have diabetes, tea may help. Oxidative stress contributes to the development of long-term complications of diabetes.

An Indian study found that tea catechins, with their strong antioxidant properties, reduce oxidative stress in diabetic red blood cells. Enjoy more

Orange juice is high in sugar, but it may still be a good beverage for people with diabetes. That's because the flavonoids in orange juice, hesperitin and naringenin, inhibit free radicals and inflammation. In animal studies, naringenin lowers cholesterol and blood sugar and helps prevent weight gain.

catechin-rich foods, like green tea, and you may protect yourself from diabetes and its complications.

Timely tips for storing and serving tea

Going green can help save the environment. When it comes to tea, going green may help save your life. Choose green tea over oolong, red, or black teas. You'll get more catechins. Follow these tips for buying, serving, and storing green tea.

- To boost absorption of green tea catechins, add some sugar and vitamin C to your tea. A splash of citrus juice — such as orange, grapefruit, lemon, or lime — should do the trick.

- Catechins break down over time. Buy only the amount of tea you'll use within six months. Jot down the purchase date on your box of tea. While the box may have a best-if-used-by date, this does not account for flavonoids — just taste.

- Store loose tea in a small, airtight container. Tea bags and foil wrappers also provide some protection.

3 ways epicatechins keep you sharp

Rev up your brain. Sharpen your wits with a cup of cocoa or a chocolate bar. Loaded with flavonoids, including catechins and epicatechins, these sweet treats may stimulate your brain.

In a Norwegian study of older people, those who regularly consumed flavonoid-rich foods, like chocolate, tea, and wine, performed better on several mental tests. For chocolate, about 10 grams — or one-third of an ounce — a day provided the maximum benefit.

A recent British study found that drinking cocoa beverages rich in flavonoids may improve performance on challenging mental tasks.

People in the study drank cocoa beverages with either 520 milligrams (mg) or 994 mg of cocoa flavonoids or a control drink. Those who drank the cocoa drinks did significantly better on a test that required them to count backward from 999 in threes. People who drank the 520 mg drink also reported less mental fatigue during the tasks.

Increase blood flow. These positive results likely stem from cocoa's ability to increase blood flow to the brain. Increased blood flow means more oxygen and nutrients for your brain cells.

In a recent study, older people drank flavonoid-rich cocoa, which contained 900 mg of epicatechins and catechins, or a cocoa lacking flavonoids for seven days. For those who drank the flavonoid-rich cocoa, blood flow to the brain increased by up to 10 percent. Surprisingly, the increase lasted for 14 days — or a week after they stopped drinking cocoa.

Another study of healthy young women reported similar results. In the University of Nottingham study, women drank a high-flavonoid cocoa drink and performed a task where they had to distinguish between vowels and consonants or odd and even numbers. Using functional magnetic resonance imaging, researchers determined which areas of the brain were activated. They noticed an increase in blood flow to the brain's gray matter for two to three hours.

How you cook your onions determines how much quercetin you get. According to a Japanese study, cooking onions in the microwave without water or frying them in oil and butter helps preserve flavonoids. But when you boil onions, you lose about 30 percent of the quercetin in the boiling water. Another way to boost your quercetin intake is to cook with onion skin. Throw some in your soups or stews, then discard it before serving, as you would a bay leaf.

Because flavonoid-rich cocoa products seem to increase blood flow and brain function, they may be helpful for older, fatigued, or sleep-deprived people. They may even be useful for treating dementia and stroke.

Get some exercise, and chocolate's benefits may be even greater. In a recent Salk Institute study, mice were given either a typical diet or a typical diet supplemented with epicatechin. Some mice ran on a wheel for two hours a day, while others remained sedentary. Then the mice were trained to find a platform in a water maze.

Mice who ate the epicatechin and exercised remembered the location of the platform longer than the other mice. They also had greater blood vessel growth in certain parts of the brain, as well as more mature brain nerve cells, indicating better communication between cells.

Genes associated with learning and memory showed an increase in activity, while genes associated with inflammation and brain degeneration were suppressed. Mice who ate epicatechin but did not exercise also showed better memory and other benefits, but not to the extent of the epicatechin and exercise group.

Unfortunately for chocolate lovers, not all chocolate has beneficial effects on your brain. For best results, look for dark chocolate rich in flavonoids.

Guard your heart. Chocolate and hearts go well together — just think of Valentine's Day. When you get a box of dark chocolates from your sweetheart, your heart also gets a sweet gift. Several studies suggest that chocolate and cocoa have heart-healthy benefits.

An observational study of the Kuna Indians, who live on the San Blas islands off the coast of Panama, provides evidence for cocoa's powers. The Kuna drink up to 40 cups of locally grown flavonoid-rich cocoa a week. Compared to people who live on mainland Panama, the Kuna had much lower risks of death from heart disease, stroke, cancer, and diabetes.

While other factors could account for the difference, the flavonoids in cocoa cannot be ruled out. In fact, further studies of the Kuna pinpointed the beneficial effects of epicatechin, including an increase in nitric oxide and blood flow.

Lab trials and other studies have found that high-flavonoid chocolate protects against LDL cholesterol oxidation, prevents platelets from clumping together, relaxes and widens blood vessels to improve blood flow, increases good HDL cholesterol, lowers blood pressure, and reduces inflammation. Mechanisms likely include a boost in nitric oxide, as well as the antioxidant and anti-inflammatory activity of cocoa flavonoids. Cocoa's positive effects on blood vessels and blood flow may be even greater among older people.

> Organic fruits and vegetables may be pricier — but they are also richer in flavonoids. One 10-year study found that organically grown tomatoes have nearly twice as many flavonoids, including quercetin and kaempferol, as those conventionally grown. Stress from pests and weather stimulates organic crops to boost their natural defense mechanisms. That means more flavonoids — and better taste.

Chocolate may even improve your chances of survival after a heart attack. In an eight-year Swedish observational study, researchers followed people who had suffered a first heart attack. Eating chocolate seemed to lower the risk of heart-related death. Those who ate chocolate less than once a month lowered their risk by 27 percent compared to those who ate none. People who ate chocolate up to once a week cut their risk by 44 percent, and those who ate chocolate twice or more weekly slashed it by 66 percent.

Here's even more evidence that a little chocolate goes a long way. An Italian study found that eating a small square of chocolate two or three times a week significantly reduces levels of C-reactive protein, a marker of inflammation. Chronic inflammation is a major risk factor for heart disease, heart attacks, and stroke.

Lower your risk of mental decline, heart attacks, and stroke with an after-dinner delight. Just sip a hot cup of cocoa or nibble a piece of dark chocolate for dessert.

Tasty tips for chocolate lovers

Chocolate will never be mistaken for a health food. But you can enjoy an occasional sweet treat while treating your body to a healthy helping of flavonoids. Keep these shopping and eating strategies in mind.

- Look past the fat. Even though dark chocolate has more fat than milk chocolate, it also has more flavonoids. In small amounts, the benefits of dark chocolate outweigh the drawbacks. Stick to 1 or 2 ounces a day.

- Darker doesn't always mean healthier. Some dark chocolate may not be as healthy as you think. That's because manufacturers often remove flavonoids because they're bitter. Instead of a health boost, you just get a large portion of fat, sugar, and calories.

- Select super sources. A recent study determined the best chocolate sources of catechins and epicatechins. Natural cocoa powder ranked first, followed by unsweetened baking chocolate, dark chocolate and semisweet baking chips, milk chocolate, and chocolate syrup.

- Rethink the milky way. A cold glass of milk seems like the perfect way to wash down your chocolate. But some studies suggest that milk impairs the absorption of cocoa flavonoids. Other experts say milk doesn't affect absorption. Stay tuned while research continues.

4 ways quercetin keeps you sharp

Protects brain cells. An apple a day doesn't just keep the doctor away. Thanks to quercetin, it can help keep your brain cells alive.

In lab tests, Canadian scientists determined that quercetin reduces the death of brain cells caused by oxidative stress and inflammation. This makes foods like apples, which contain quercetin, potential weapons against mental decline and brain disorders like Parkinson's disease.

Parkinson's disease involves the loss of dopaminergic neurons, or brain cells that provide the neurotransmitter dopamine. By lowering oxidative stress and inflammation, quercetin may help safeguard these important brain cells.

Quercetin-rich foods	
1 sweet onion	48.99 mg*
1 medium red onion	36.77 mg
1 medium onion	23.56 mg
1 cup chopped scallions	18.33 mg
1 medium pear	8.03 mg
1 medium apple, with skin	7.77 mg
1 cup green tea	6.38 mg
1 cup black tea	4.72 mg

* milligrams

Boosts memory. When you think of apple juice, perhaps you think of juice boxes and sippy cups. But apple juice is not just for kids. For a better memory in your golden years, try sipping more of this "childhood" drink.

A series of animal studies by University of Massachusetts, Lowell researchers showcases the potential brain-boosting power of apple juice.

- Apple juice helps maintain acetylcholine levels in aging mice. Acetylcholine, a key neurotransmitter, is required for a good memory, and low levels of acetylcholine have been linked to Alzheimer's disease. Not surprisingly, the aging mice who got apple juice also performed better on maze tests.

- Mice who received the equivalent of two glasses of apple juice a day for a month produced less beta-amyloid, the protein responsible for forming plaques in the brains of people with Alzheimer's disease.

- Aging mice whose diet included apple juice did much better on maze tests and had less oxidative brain damage than mice given a standard diet. Mice were given the human equivalent of two to three cups of apple juice or two to four apples a day.

Antioxidants, including quercetin and other flavonoids, in apples and apple juice get the credit. In one Cornell University study of rats, quercetin seemed to protect brain cells from oxidative stress, which has been linked to Alzheimer's disease and other brain disorders.

Maximizes mitochondria. Little things can make a big difference. Take mitochondria, for example. These tiny powerhouses within your cells burn food for energy. But over time, damage caused by free radicals can weaken mitochondria — and weakened mitochondria can lead to diseases, including Parkinson's disease and Alzheimer's disease.

Studies show quercetin has a positive effect on mitochondria. University of South Carolina researchers found that quercetin boosted mitochondria in both the brain and muscles of mice. The mice had better endurance on treadmill tests and were spontaneously more active, choosing to spend more time running on a wheel. Researchers noted that the brain plays an important role in exercise. Motivation and mood can be affected by brain metabolism, and increased mitochondrial activity can enhance this metabolism.

> Other flavonoids also protect your health. Kaempferol, a flavonoid found in tea, broccoli, grapefruit, and other plant sources, may reduce the risk of heart disease and ovarian cancer.

Quercetin also boosted endurance in college students. Twelve students, who were not regular workout warriors, drank Tang containing 500 milligrams of quercetin for seven days. After a week of quercetin supplementation, they were able to ride a stationary bike 13 percent longer before becoming too tired to continue.

Hampers heart disease. Take care of your heart, and you'll also take care of your brain. Heart disease and its risk factors may increase your risk for dementia — not to mention a heart attack or stroke.

Several studies suggest that quercetin can help your heart. A Finnish study found that a higher quercetin intake — mostly from apples and onions — lowers the risk of death from heart disease. Eating more quercetin-rich foods may also reduce the risk of type 2 diabetes. A study of flavonoids and specific food sources found that apples lower heart disease risk in women.

Quercetin supplements helped lower blood pressure in people with high blood pressure. A pair of Dutch studies suggest quercetin lowers the risk of heart attack and stroke.

Obesity can boost your risk of heart disease, diabetes, and dementia. In lab tests involving fat cells, University of Georgia researchers found that quercetin — especially when combined with resveratrol — has powerful anti-obesity effects.

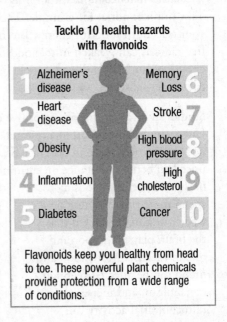

Tackle 10 health hazards with flavonoids

1 Alzheimer's disease
2 Heart disease
3 Obesity
4 Inflammation
5 Diabetes
6 Memory Loss
7 Stroke
8 High blood pressure
9 High cholesterol
10 Cancer

Flavonoids keep you healthy from head to toe. These powerful plant chemicals provide protection from a wide range of conditions.

Bite into an apple for brain-boosting boron

Quercetin isn't the only reason to eat apples. Apples are also one of the top sources of boron in the American diet. Boron, a trace mineral that protects your bones and joints, may also keep your brain young.

Researchers in North Dakota have been working to find out how boron affects your brain. In a series of studies, older men and women ate either a diet with too little boron or one with plenty. People who didn't get enough boron scored poorly on tests of brain function, including hand-eye coordination, manual dexterity, attention, and memory. To keep these important skills well into your golden years, be sure you eat this delicious food each day.

As a supplement, quercetin may help relieve allergy symptoms by controlling the release of histamine. Pair it with vitamin C to maximize its impact. Supplemental quercetin also shows promise as an immunity booster. The antioxidant binds to viruses and prevents them from reproducing. In studies of soldiers and cyclists, quercetin reduced the number of colds and sore throats.

Other good sources of boron include peanut butter, wine, raisins, and peanuts. You can also get boron from coffee, milk, potatoes, beans, peaches, bananas, and fruit juices.

High doses come with higher risk

Eat all the flavonoid-rich foods you want. But keep in mind that high doses of flavonoids from supplements may not be as safe.

For example, high doses of quercetin may cause nausea, headache, and tingling of your extremities. When taken intravenously, it may also cause vomiting, sweating, flushing, difficulty breathing, and even kidney toxicity.

At high doses, green tea extract may trigger nausea, vomiting, abdominal pain, and diarrhea. Other unpleasant effects, such as agitation, restlessness, insomnia, tremors, dizziness, and confusion may be due to the caffeine in green tea rather than its flavonoids.

Because flavonoids stop platelets from clumping, high doses may increase your risk of bleeding if taken with blood-thinning drugs like warfarin, Plavix, and nonsteroidal anti-inflammatory drugs (NSAIDs), which include aspirin and ibuprofen. Other drug interactions can occur with grapefruit juice. High doses of the flavonoids naringenin, quercetin, and EGCG may also interfere with certain medications.

Flavonoids inhibit the absorption of nonheme iron, the kind found in plants and many iron supplements. To maximize your iron absorption, avoid high-flavonoid beverages or supplements during mealtimes.

Folate

leafy green vegetables • legumes • citrus fruits • liver • enriched cereals • enriched grains and pasta

Many people use the terms folate and folic acid interchangeably, and even though they both refer to the same, very important B vitamin, they indicate different forms.

- Folate occurs naturally in foods.

- Folic acid is a synthetic version used in vitamin supplements and to fortify foods, like breads and cereals.

However you get it, this B vitamin is crucial to good health. Besides working like an antioxidant to ward off destructive attacks from free radicals, folate also helps your body form red blood cells and produce DNA, the genetic building blocks of your body.

Since 1998, the U.S. and Canadian governments have required food manufacturers to add folic acid to grain products. This came after it was discovered a folate deficiency was behind neural tube defects, a type of birth defect affecting babies' brains and spines. This fortification means most people get at least 100 micrograms (mcg) of folic acid every day.

Surprisingly, that's not enough. Since folate is water soluble, your body can't store it. You need a continual supply from your diet or supplements to maintain healthy levels. The recommended amount is 400 mcg a day.

Certain medications and medical conditions, like celiac disease, can keep your body from absorbing folate — causing a deficiency. You may not notice any symptoms at first, but inside your body, things won't be going well.

3/4 cup Total whole-grain cereal	676 mcg*
1 cup cooked enriched white rice	238 mcg
1/2 cup cooked lentils	179 mcg
10 pretzels	172 mcg
1 cup cooked broccoli	168 mcg
1 cup cooked enriched pasta	167 mcg
1/2 cup cooked spinach	132 mcg
1 cup orange juice from frozen concentrate	110 mcg

* micrograms

Blood cells won't divide properly resulting in megaloblastic anemia, a condition where fewer, larger red blood cells can't circulate enough oxygen. Eventually, you'll start to feel tired, weak, and short of breath.

Perhaps most important to your heart and brain is the critical relationship between folate and homocysteine. Homocysteine is a bad guy in the world of health. This amino acid damages blood cells and increases your risk of dangerous clots.

Because of this, high levels of homocysteine are linked to both heart disease and dementia. It forms when your body breaks down certain compounds. Normally, it's converted into other, beneficial amino acids, but that process requires folate. In other words, you need folate to turn homocysteine into something less dangerous. It's been proven too little folate in your blood means too much homocysteine, and vice versa.

Cereal (without milk)	% Daily Value of folic acid
1 cup Kellogg's Special K	100%
1 cup Kellogg's Product 19	100%
1 cup General Mills Cheerios	50%
3/4 cup General Mills Wheaties	50%
1/2 cup Post Grape-Nuts	50%
1 cup Post Raisin Bran	50%
1 cup Kellogg's Raisin Bran	25%
3/4 cup Kellogg's Frosted Flakes	25%
1 cup Post Shredded Wheat	4%

4 ways folate keeps you sharp

Helps you stay on the ball. Folate is unquestionably related to strong brainpower and memory, perhaps because of antioxidant properties or its link to homocysteine.

In a 10-year study of more than 13,000 older women, those who ate the most green leafy vegetables, like spinach and romaine lettuce, scored better on memory and mental sharpness tests when they were in their 70s. And a recent Korean study found that people with a folate deficiency were three and a half times more likely to develop dementia.

Too little folate means more homocysteine in your blood. Besides the fact that homocysteine can damage the blood vessels in your brain, it's also connected to deterioration of the hippocampus, an area of your brain essential to memory. Getting extra folate may help your brain work better and faster by controlling the amount of homocysteine.

All in all, this is definitely one supplement you should take if you want to help prevent age-related memory loss.

Slashes your risk of stroke. A stroke can wreak havoc on your brain, affecting everything from speech to thought processes to memory. How incredible that you can lower your risk by 18 percent with one supplement. A major review of eight studies confirmed that taking anywhere from 500 micrograms (mcg) to 15,000 mcg of folic acid a day gave this kind of protection.

If that doesn't convince you, consider this. Since folic acid fortification became mandatory in 1998, fewer people have died from strokes in the United States and Canada.

It all comes back to homocysteine — the damage it does to your blood vessels, how it thickens and narrows your arteries, and how it increases your likelihood of clots. Lowering homocysteine means a lower risk of stroke, and you can lower homocysteine by eating foods rich in folate or by taking folic acid supplements.

> Folate was first identified in spinach leaves, so it seemed only appropriate to name it from the Latin word for leaf — *folium*. That should help you remember leafy greens are a great source of folate.

Helps lower your BP. High blood pressure means less oxygen gets to your brain and you carry a greater risk of stroke, two situations that spell trouble for sharp thinking. A combined study followed over 150,000 women for eight years to see how folate affected their blood pressure. Women in their 30s and 40s cut their risk of high blood pressure almost in half when they got 1,000 mcg of folate a day from both food and supplements. Women over age 50 showed less of a benefit, but they still cut their risk by 18 percent.

No explanation is definite, but researchers think folate helps your blood pressure by interacting with nitric oxide, a hormone vitally important to your heart health. Cells lining the inside of your blood vessels — called endothelial cells — naturally release nitric oxide, which, in turn, helps keep your blood vessels relaxed and flexible.

Supple, wide-open blood vessels make it possible for your blood to flow smoothly. The older you get, the less nitric oxide your cells produce and the less flexible your blood vessels become. Extra folate rushes to the rescue by helping your endothelial cells make more nitric oxide.

> Three researchers won the 1998 Nobel Prize in Medicine for their discovery recognizing nitric oxide (NO) as an important chemical messenger in the cardio-vascular system. NO also plays a vital role in memory, learning, and regulating your sleep-wake cycle.

Keeps your hearing sharp and your eyesight keen. Foods full of folate — everything from green leafy vegetables to the surprisingly folate-rich orange — can help keep your senses in peak form.

- Want to throw out your hearing aid? A brand new study showed that men over age 60 who had a high intake of folate from foods and supplements were 20 percent less likely to develop hearing loss. There's no official explanation, but folate's antioxidant properties may help protect your ear's delicate inner workings. Older research points out folic acid supplements protected low-frequency hearing the most.

- Folate, along with other B vitamins, proved in an important 2009 study it can protect women from age-related macular degeneration (AMD). Those who took B-vitamin supplements daily — 2.5 milligrams (mg) of folic acid, 50 mg of vitamin B6, and 1 mg of vitamin B12 — for seven years were up to 40 percent less likely to develop AMD.

The researchers explain it this way. If folate eliminates homocysteine, it can't damage the lining of your blood vessels, including those in your eyes. And, as an anti-oxidant, folate protects the eyes' fragile photoreceptors crucial for sharp vision.

Smart shoppers know their DFEs

Folic acid is the synthetic form of folate. It's used in dietary supplements and added to breads, cereals, and other grain products. Researchers say it's more readily absorbed into your bloodstream than folate, which occurs naturally in food. That means, as far as your body is concerned, 1 microgram (mcg) of folate from spinach is not exactly equal to 1 mcg of folic acid from enriched pasta. That's why the Food and Nutrition Board of the Institute of Medicine introduced the Dietary Folate Equivalent (DFE).

> Your body may not thoroughly absorb folate if you take aspirin or antacids on a regular basis. Talk to your doctor about testing your folate levels if you take these drugs often.

They've determined you would have to eat 1.7 mcg of food folate to absorb the same amount as in 1 mcg of folic acid. To avoid confusion, this new unit, the DFE, will do the math for you. It converts all forms of folate into a standardized unit.

Here are a couple of points to keep in mind.

- You absorb more of the vitamin if you take a folic acid supplement on an empty stomach than if you take it with food.

- Watch out for labels that still use micrograms instead of DFE.

Folate: cancer risk or remedy?

There's a storm brewing over supplemental folic acid and colon cancer, but like most issues, there are two sides to the story.

Companies began fortifying foods with folic acid back in 1998. Soon after, doctors noticed about a 100 percent increase in blood levels of folic acid. About the same time, the number of colon cancer cases started to increase, and they've been on the rise ever since. Those who think they are related make these points:

> Before the United States required grain products to be fortified with folic acid, 26 percent of the population didn't get the minimum requirement. Today, less than 1 percent are deficient.

- One of the main functions of folate in your body is to create new cells. Some experts believe this means it could stimulate pre-cancerous and cancerous cells to grow and reproduce. That means a high intake of folic acid could turn colon adenomas, or benign tumors, into cancers and small cancers into larger ones.

- Folic acid seems to impair your cancer immune defenses by reducing the number of natural killer cells in your body.

Here's the other side to the story.

- Folic acid doesn't appear to create cancer where there isn't any to start with.

- Long-term, high doses of folic acid are proven to protect against colon cancer. A recent Korean study found that women were two-thirds less likely to develop colon cancer when they took folic acid supplements.

The bottom line is there's no absolute evidence that one causes the other, but you can take precautions. Up to half the United States population over age 50 has one or more benign colon tumors. Most of these don't cause symptoms, but they are precursors to colon cancer. If you've been diagnosed with a colon adenoma, don't get extra folic acid through a multivitamin or enriched foods.

Most experts agree it's nearly impossible to get too much folate from vegetables and other natural sources.

> People in Greece, following the traditional, vegetable-rich Mediterranean diet, get an average of 559 micrograms of folate every day.

Garlic

acts as an antioxidant • lowers blood pressure • prevents blood clots • reduces cholesterol • fights infections • battles Alzheimer's disease • boosts energy

Garlic does more than add a rich aroma and biting flavor to foods. It brings specific, healthy elements, called organosulfur compounds, to the table, as well. All you have to do is release these little superstars so they can get to work.

Within 10 to 60 seconds of crushing a clove of garlic, a cascade of chemical reactions produces probably the most well-known organosulfur compound, allicin. It's so remarkably beneficial, the World Health Organization recommends getting about 2 to 5 milligrams (mg) of it a day. That's easy to do since one garlic clove contains anywhere from 5 to 18 mg of allicin. Just think, every time you sprinkle, dice, squeeze, chew, or mash garlic, you're giving your body a powerful shot of natural disease-fighters.

Eating a clove of garlic every day is the no-fuss way to get allicin. Unfortunately, some people can't tolerate the strong taste, and it isn't always easy to add it to your menu. That's when you might turn to supplements. Most studies on garlic use tablets of dried garlic powder or aged garlic extract (AGE), and sometimes garlic oil.

Just remember, all supplements are not created equal. Most are not standardized and the amount of organosulfur compounds can vary wildly depending on how the garlic is processed. Unless you consult an independent testing firm like ConsumerLab.com — at *www.consumerlab.com* — you just have to hope you're getting what you pay for.

Exactly how allicin works in your body is not fully understood, perhaps because researchers are not able to track it through the bloodstream. Even after people ate 25 grams of fresh garlic — anywhere from six to 13 cloves — scientists could not detect any allicin in their blood. This suggests it is absorbed into your body quite rapidly.

> The last thing you want is garlic breath, but some day you may be brushing your teeth or gargling with products containing garlic extract. The antibacterial properties of this tasty herb can really do a number on the major bacteria that cause cavities.

6 ways garlic keeps you sharp

Brings down your BP. The higher your blood pressure, the more likely it is garlic will help lower it. After examining the results of 11 studies, experts confirmed garlic supplements were as helpful as beta-blockers and ACE inhibitors in reducing blood pressure numbers. The allicin from garlic is believed to encourage your blood vessels to produce nitric oxide, a chemical that relaxes and dilates the vessels, allowing blood to flow more easily. This ensures your brain gets plenty of life-giving oxygen and nutrients. Most studies used about the amount of allicin you would find in one clove of garlic. Talk to your doctor before supplementing with garlic if you are already taking medication to lower your blood pressure.

Banishes blood clots. Cut your finger and you soon realize clotting outside your body is a good thing. Blood clots inside your body, on the other hand, spell danger, often in the form of heart attacks and brain-damaging strokes. Many elements in garlic work together to discourage your blood from clotting in the first place and to boost fibrinolysis, your body's natural process that keeps blood clots from growing and causing problems.

Challenges high cholesterol. It's a mixed bag of study results, which means for every piece of research you find singing the praises of garlic for high cholesterol, you'll find one that declares it ineffective. Generally, the opinion is you could modestly lower your total cholesterol, LDL cholesterol, and triglycerides with garlic for the short-term. Don't expect miracles and don't think this will cure you of high cholesterol forever. But if you want to drop your numbers a tad or add to an existing cholesterol-lowering regimen, extra garlic in your diet may be just the ticket.

> Could it be garlic fights colds by keeping people so far away from you they can't infect you with their germs?

Fights off infections. Your grannie may have hung garlic around her neck to ward off colds, but all you really have to do to give your immune system a kick in the pants is eat it. Garlic is loaded with compounds that fight both bacterial and viral infections, often making it less likely you'll get a cold and helping you recover faster if you get one.

Gives aid against Alzheimer's. Aged garlic extract (AGE) is already known to protect your brain by shielding nerve cells from toxins, encouraging the healthy growth of nerve tissue, and safeguarding brainpower and memory by acting as an antioxidant.

Now, a recent study out of India finds garlic may delay or even prevent Alzheimer's disease. Researchers believe it's the various organosulfur compounds in AGE that keep amyloid plaques from forming.

These tangles of hardened proteins between nerve cells in your brain are one of the characteristics of Alzheimer's disease.

Powers you up. You may have heard the story that ancient Egyptian slaves and Roman soldiers were fed garlic to keep them energized. A recent Japanese study bears this out. Researchers found:

- AGE helps specific muscles metabolize blood sugar more easily during exercise, producing extra energy.

- garlic boosts nitric oxide production, widening your blood vessels and allowing more oxygen to flow to fatigued muscles.

- AGE works as an antioxidant to fight dangerous free radicals produced during exercise.

Kitchen secrets lock in benefits

It's fun and healthy to make garlic part of your daily menu — but not if you cook all the valuable properties away. Here's expert advice on how to get the most out of your cloves.

- Heating garlic in any way reduces its clot-busting power, but if you can keep cooking time to under three minutes, you'll preserve more benefits.

- Fresh, crushed garlic retains more of the healthful organosulfur compound, allicin, than preserved types of garlic, and it has more potent heart-healthy effects than dried garlic.

- Garlic keeps its antioxidant power after most cooking methods.

> Garlic is a member of the lily family, so if you are allergic to flowers like hyacinths or tulips, you may also react to garlic.

Garlic's hidden danger

Garlic is very safe if you eat it in a normal diet, and supplements in recommended doses are safe for most people. However, if you are taking any kind of prescription blood thinner, like warfarin (Coumadin), or another supplement known to increase bleeding, like ginkgo biloba, extra garlic could be dangerous for you. Because garlic interferes with your blood's natural ability to clot, it could also cause problems if you have a bleeding disorder or you are having a surgical or dental procedure.

> Chopped garlic is great for your health but not so much fun to smell on your fingers. Get rid of the lingering odor by rubbing your fingers on your stainless steel sink or a stainless steel utensil.

Ginseng

controls blood sugar • cuts down on colds • boosts flu shot • fights fatigue • provides antioxidant power

You can buy it as a tablet, capsule, extract, root, or tea. Perhaps you down it in an energy drink or rub it on in a cream. However you "do" ginseng, you're joining the millions of people worldwide who believe in the healing powers of this ancient herb.

Ginseng is a flowering plant that grows best in the shade. It has red berries and a famous, yellow-brown root shaped something like a human body. In fact, its Chinese name translates as "man-root." Its Greek botanical name, panax, means "cure-all," probably because it was historically used to heal many different conditions — everything from allergies to wrinkles. Today's experts won't call ginseng a cure-all, but there's proof it's a safe, natural addition to your home-remedy arsenal.

The ginseng root is especially rich in ginsenosides, chemical compounds believed responsible for its healing powers. And although the root is most widely tested and marketed, the ginseng berries and leaves are also beneficial.

Many factors affect how potent ginseng is, including:

- the plant species.
- what kind of soil it was grown in.
- how old the plant was when harvested.
- what time of year it was harvested.
- what country it was grown in.
- whether it was grown wild or field-farmed.
- how the plant was processed.

Natural Ginsenoside Levels

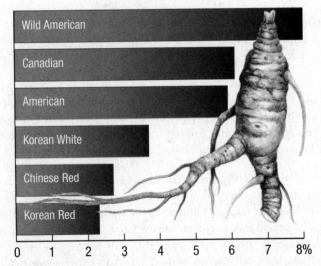

4 ways ginseng keeps you sharp

Manages your blood sugar. Ginseng could be a safe addition to your therapy if you have diabetes. Research shows it can lower blood sugar levels without causing a dangerous drop. In addition, the herb seems to work directly on your pancreas, increasing insulin production and reducing insulin resistance. Shop carefully since American ginseng and Korean red ginseng were the only two types shown in studies to lower blood sugar, while Asian (panax) ginseng can actually raise it. Remember to only take this supplement with your doctor's knowledge and approval.

A 14-week study of more than 250 middle-age volunteers showed those taking an herbal combination of ginkgo and *Panax ginseng* scored better on memory tests than those taking a placebo.

Strengthens your immune system. Get a little boost during cold and flu season with a ginseng supplement. It can:

- trigger your body to produce more T-cells, a type of white blood cell that seeks out and destroys bacteria and viruses.

- add extra power to any antibiotics you might be taking for a bacterial infection.

- give your flu shot a little added oomph.

Many people swear their daily dose of ginseng means shorter and fewer colds than usual.

Picks you up. Try ginseng for added energy and see if it works for you. Even though the clinical evidence is not rock-solid, athletes in China have used it for decades, believing it enhances their performance. One eight-week study on people between the ages of 40 and 70 found those taking 400 milligrams of ginseng a day had faster reaction times than the others. You may find ginseng helps you feel less fatigued or a little more on the ball.

Unleashes antioxidants. The ginsenosides in ginseng give the herb some antioxidant power, making it useful in the fight against high cholesterol, memory loss, high blood pressure, and many other conditions where dangerous free radicals cause damage.

The largest farmed seven-year-old American ginseng root weighed over 2 pounds. This might bring up to $35 in today's market. A 2-pound wild root could sell for $300 or more.

Dosing hints guarantee more bang for your buck

Read the label on any ginseng product before you buy to see exactly what you're getting. It should tell you the type of ginseng, what part of the plant was used, whether it contains powder or extract, and what amount of ginsenosides is in the final product.

Type	Recommended amount of ginsenosides in product		Daily dose	Amount of ginseno-sides in daily dose
	% total ginsenosides	Ginsenosides per gram of ginseng		
Asian ginseng root powder	1.5%	15 mg	1,000-2,000 mg	15-30 mg
American ginseng root powder	2%	20 mg	1,000-2,000 mg	20-40 mg
Asian ginseng extract	3%	30 mg	200 mg in two 100-mg doses	6 mg
American ginseng extract	4%	40 mg	200 mg in two 100-mg doses	8 mg

Get smart on label lingo

Asian ginseng *(Panax ginseng)* is mostly grown in China, Korea, and Russia, but it's nearly extinct in the wild. This is the type most often used in research.

American ginseng *(Panax quinquefolius)* is native to North America — mainly southeastern Canada and cool, temperate parts of the United States — but is also grown in China. It's especially prized because its roots have more natural ginsenosides than the Asian varieties. Thousands of pounds of American ginseng are exported every year, mostly to Asian countries.

Siberian ginseng contains no ginsenosides and is not considered a true ginseng.

Wild ginseng is not planted or farmed in any way, but it's simply harvested from wherever it grows naturally. Both American and Asian ginseng grow wild, but only in specific northern areas of North America and China. Because it contains higher levels of ginsenosides than field-farmed ginseng, wild ginseng is highly demanded, highly priced, overharvested, and now endangered.

> Talk to your doctor before trying ginseng if you are taking a blood thinner like warfarin (Coumadin). Ginseng can affect clotting.

Field-cultivated or field-farmed ginseng is grown in tilled beds under artificial shade. It can be harvested after just five to seven years, but it brings a much lower price than wild ginseng.

White ginseng is unprocessed and air-dried.

Red ginseng always comes from cultivated roots, usually grown in China or South Korea. They are left unpeeled, then steamed and sun-dried, resulting in a red-brown color. This process is said to keep the ginsenosides from breaking down, creating a more potent product.

Grape seed extract

lowers blood pressure • protects brain cells from damage
• encourages good circulation • cuts heart disease
risk for diabetes sufferers

Grape juice and wine may combine all the goodness found in the
grape skin, pulp, and seeds, but don't overlook a concentrated extract
you get by crushing just the seeds. These tiny pips are a rich store-
house of fatty acids and natural
plant chemicals, containing
even more vitamin E,
flavonoids, linoleic acid, and
antioxidant compounds than
grape skin. The resulting grape
seed extract (GSE) is used to
fight a number of diseases.

> Grapes are full of other good-
> for-you ingredients, many of
> which are discussed in the
> *Flavonoids* and *Resveratrol*
> chapters.

The specific antioxidants in GSE are called oligomeric proantho-
cyanidin complexes (OPCs). Early lab studies show OPCs act like
any other anti-oxidant, protecting against free radical damage.

Sold as pills, capsules, and a liquid, look for GSE that is
standardized to an OPC content of at least 95 percent or is 40 to
80 percent proanthocyanidins.

4 ways GSE keeps you sharp

Halts high blood pressure. A month-long study at the University of
California, Davis showed grape seed extract (GSE) lowers blood
pressure. Researchers tested people with a combination of health
risk factors known as metabolic syndrome — insulin resistance,
belly fat, troublesome cholesterol levels, and high blood pressure.

All those taking GSE, whether at 150 milligrams (mg) or 300 mg a day, significantly dropped their blood pressure numbers.

It works by encouraging the cells along the inside walls of your blood vessels to produce more nitric oxide, a chemical messenger that keeps the blood vessels relaxed and dilated. Blood flows more quickly and easily through blood vessels that are flexible and wide open, reducing your risk of heart disease and ensuring oxygen-rich blood gets to your brain.

Talk to your doctor before starting GSE if you have high blood pressure. You don't want this supplement interacting with other medications or lowering your blood pressure too much.

Prevents damage to brain cells. In animal and lab studies, GSE's success in fighting one distinctive feature of Alzheimer's disease (AD) gives scientists hope it could some day be a significant weapon against this tragic condition. It all starts with protein.

Proteins exist inside every cell of every living organism. They allow your body to do all the things it must to stay alive, like break down food to power your muscles, send signals through your brain, and carry nutrients through your blood. All proteins are made of a long chain of amino acids joined together like a string of beads. They begin life in this long form, but in order to function properly, each protein must fold up into a three-dimensional shape, one where different amino acids within the chain join to others. There are thousands of different proteins, each with its own function and final shape.

Sometimes, for reasons not fully understood, proteins in healthy brain cells do not fold correctly. This "misfolding" leads to a buildup and clumping of proteins in the tissue between your brain's neurons. The neurons lose connection with each other, they die, and brain tissue shrinks. This damage is a telltale sign of AD.

Certain natural chemicals in GSE may stop proteins from misfolding. When mice with AD were given grape seed extract for five months, they showed a significant decrease in protein buildup.

They had best results when the mice were given lower doses of GSE over a longer period of time. Tests on people are next.

Promotes better blood flow. There's good, solid research that GSE can help with a painful condition called chronic venous insufficiency, where the veins in your legs have trouble sending blood back to your heart. The blood ends up pooling in your legs causing swelling and fatigue. In several studies, GSE fought swelling and other symptoms, and encouraged better circulation. This natural remedy acted faster and gave longer relief than other treatments.

Decreases heart disease risk. A four-week study of people suffering from type 2 diabetes showed grape seed extract reduced their risk of heart disease. After receiving 600 milligrams of GSE every day, they had improved in three cardiac danger zones — fewer markers of body-wide inflammation, less cellular damage from free radicals, and lower levels of blood sugar.

Grape seed offers healthy oil change

Grape seed oil is good for you both inside and out. Try it for a heaping helping of wholesome nutrients and a light, fruity taste.

Extracted from the seeds of grapes, it's usually a byproduct of the winemaking process. There are a few sources in the United States, but it's mainly imported from France, Switzerland, or Italy.

In the kitchen, grape seed oil is perfect for the frying pan because of its high smoke point. That means you can really kick up the heat without it breaking down and losing both flavor and nutrition. It blends well with other ingredients so try it in dressings, marinades, or other recipes.

And because it's an excellent source of vitamin E and good-for-you unsaturated fats, you might be tempted to really pour it on. But be careful — grape seed oil is also high in omega-6 fatty acids. These aren't necessarily unhealthy fats, but most people eating a Western diet full of fried and fast foods get way too much of them. So don't use grape seed oil instead of other healthy choices, like olive oil. Just let it be a small part of a nutritious diet.

There's not much scientific research on the subject, but because of its antioxidant properties, you may also find grape seed oil used in massage or as an ingredient in skin products.

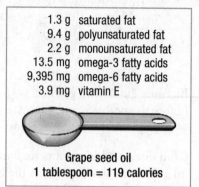

1.3 g	saturated fat
9.4 g	polyunsaturated fat
2.2 g	monounsaturated fat
13.5 mg	omega-3 fatty acids
9,395 mg	omega-6 fatty acids
3.9 mg	vitamin E

Grape seed oil
1 tablespoon = 119 calories

Get clued in on bleeding risk

Grape seed extract (GSE), like all dietary supplements, is not regulated in any way, so you want to buy from a reputable manufacturer. Even then, there's no guarantee every batch will contain the same amount of active ingredients.

That being said, GSE is reported to be a fairly safe supplement for most people. There weren't a lot of side effects in clinical trials, and experts have recommended doses up to 450 milligrams a day for as long as 12 weeks.

GSE could be dangerous if you have a bleeding disorder or are currently taking medicine to thin your blood — warfarin (Coumadin) or a nonsteroidal anti-inflammatory, like aspirin. Because of its affect on your blood's ability to clot, stop using GSE a few weeks before any kind of surgery or dental procedure.

Gum disease

red, swollen, or tender gums • bleeding while
brushing or flossing • receding gums • loose teeth
• mouth sores • chronic bad breath

Bleeding gums are a big deal — a sure sign something is wrong.
Ignore the problem and you may find out how not taking care of
your teeth and gums can rob you of your memories.

Gum disease, also called periodontal disease (PD), is a chronic
infection that develops when the bacteria in your mouth settle in
and grow on your teeth and gums. Gingivitis is the mildest form.
Your only symptoms may be gums that are red, swollen, and bleed
easily. It's fairly simple to reverse the damage at this stage with a
little extra TLC from you and your dentist.

But if left untreated, the infection can spread below your gums and
into the bones supporting your teeth. This more serious condition
is called periodontitis. Your gums begin to pull away from your
teeth forming little pockets that become infected, you can develop
sores in your mouth, and your teeth become loose or don't fit
together as they used to. At this point, you should see a specialist.
Periodontists have extra training and are up on the latest
techniques for treating the disease.

Although bacteria starts the PD ball rolling, other things influence
how severe and widespread it will be.

- Genetics. You might be among the 30 percent of people
  who carry a certain gene making you more likely to develop
  PD — even if you take excellent care of your teeth.

- Hormones. Changes like those experienced during
  menopause can affect your gums, making them more
  sensitive and vulnerable to disease.

- Smoking. In addition to the many unhealthy consequences of smoking, the chemicals in tobacco cause you to heal more slowly, prolonging the cycle of inflammation. They also interfere with the success of many PD treatments.

Perhaps the most important thing to understand about gum disease is how it can impact your overall health. Once the bacteria in your mouth enters your bloodstream, it can travel everywhere. In addition, the ongoing inflammation behind gum disease triggers an inflammatory response throughout your body. Although inflammation is usually a good thing — a natural way of fighting infection and healing injuries — it's bad news if it goes on too long. Here's how gum disease is linked to two very threatening chronic conditions.

Heart disease. Suffer from gum disease and you are almost twice as likely as others to develop heart disease. It can also make any existing heart condition worse. There are more than 50 clinical studies linking these two conditions and several theories explaining what may be happening.

- Your body's killer cells can't tell the difference between certain proteins in the bacteria triggering gum disease and similar good proteins your body makes and uses. When they attack

Have you just shed a few pounds? Then smile, your teeth and gums are healthier for it. Research shows people who are considered obese — having a Body Mass Index (BMI) over 30 — are twice as likely to develop gum disease, probably due to body-wide inflammation and insulin resistance, which means insulin has trouble moving glucose into receptor cells where it can be used.

Visit the National Heart Lung and Blood Institute's website at *www.nhlbisupport.com/bmi* to calculate your BMI. If you're in the danger zone, do what you can to lose weight and take extra care of your teeth.

this second kind of protein, they cause damage to your arteries.

- When the bacteria from your mouth enters your bloodstream, it attaches to fatty plaques inside your heart's blood vessels. This thickens the blood vessel walls and causes clots to form.

- The inflammation caused by gum disease spreads throughout your body and produces swelling in your arteries. This leads to reduced blood flow and even more damage.

The good news is that treating your gum disease and eliminating periodontal bacteria reduces the buildup of plaque in your arteries and lowers your risk of atherosclerosis.

Alzheimer's disease. Inflammation within your brain is a critical part of Alzheimer's disease (AD). Many experts believe anything like PD that sets off body-wide inflammation also triggers it in your brain. A study of twins supports this theory. Those exposed to systemic inflammation by middle age quadrupled their risk of developing AD later in life. Others think the bacteria sparking gum disease is able to spread to your brain, causing it to respond with inflammation.

More and more research is proving how gum disease is connected to other dangerous conditions. That means keeping your teeth and gums healthy is more important than ever. Even though the American Academy of Periodontology says about three out of four Americans suffer from some kind of gum disease, only 3 percent get treatment.

> Periodontal disease is the number-one cause of tooth loss.

Because it is an infection, you'd think antibiotics would be the best choice of treatment. But overusing antibiotics increases the risk of developing antibiotic-resistant strains of bacteria. There are several surgical and nonsurgical procedures your periodontist may suggest, and those may be right for you. But you must start making healthy choices now to keep gum disease at bay.

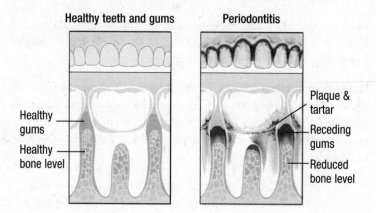

Healthy teeth and gums

Healthy gums

Healthy bone level

Periodontitis

Plaque & tartar

Receding gums

Reduced bone level

3 tactics to fight gum disease

Practice good dental hygiene. The best way to prevent gum disease is to keep your mouth clean and free of decay-causing bacteria. That means a daily routine of oral care and twice-a-year visits to your dentist. Here are tips from the American Dental Association (ADA) on the best way to clean your teeth and gums.

- Brush twice a day with a soft-bristled toothbrush. Pick one that fits your mouth and lets you reach all areas. Clean behind the surfaces of your front teeth.

- Don't forget your tongue. Brush it gently to get rid of bacteria and freshen your breath.

- Choose a fluoride toothpaste to protect your teeth from decay.

- Floss once a day to remove plaque from areas your toothbrush can't reach.

- Swish a couple of times a day. Antimicrobial mouthwashes help kill bacteria, while fluoride rinses prevent tooth decay.

Look for the ADA Seal of Acceptance on any dental product before you buy, indicating the ADA Council on Scientific Affairs has evaluated it for safety and effectiveness.

Make smart nutrition choices. Eating healthy is a natural defense against gum disease. Start with two easy changes — limit sweets that feed the bacteria in your mouth, and drink lots of water to help create more saliva and wash away plaque. Here are a few other things to consider.

- Vitamin C. It's a powerful antioxidant that helps restore collagen, the main protein in connective tissue. To someone suffering from PD, that means it helps heal sores in your mouth, strengthens gum tissue, and repairs tiny blood vessels. Eat a couple of grapefruit a day and you'll get about 180 milligrams of vitamin C. Research shows this amount lessens bleeding from your gums if you already suffer from PD and reduces your risk of developing the disease in the first place.

> According to the American Academy of Periodontology, the amount of gum tissue in your mouth is equal to the amount of skin on your arm from your wrist to your elbow. If this area was red and swollen, you would see a doctor. Treat gum disease just as seriously.

- Cranberries. Certain elements in this tart favorite keep bacteria from sticking to the surface of your teeth, making it harder for them to grow and cause problems. If that's not enough, every cup of unsweetened cranberry juice is loaded with vitamin C.

- Green tea. Catechins are natural chemicals in green tea leaves that act as an antioxidant to fight inflammation and reduce symptoms of PD. Drink it regularly and do your gums a favor.

> Take a short quiz at The American Academy of Periodontology's website, www.perio.org/consumer/4 a.html#, to find out your risk of developing gum disease.

- Omega-3 fatty acids. A five-year study out of Japan found the anti-inflammatory properties of fish oil slowed the development of periodontal disease (PD).

- Dairy foods. It may be the lactic acid in foods like milk, cheese, and yogurt, or it could be the calcium that is so beneficial. Whatever the reason, studies show getting plenty of dairy every day protects you from gum disease.

- Whole grains. These high-fiber foods are all about controlling inflammation — most likely by lowering the levels of sugar in your blood and improving insulin sensitivity. At least four servings a day of whole-grain bread, cereal, brown rice, bran, and other grains may mean no PD for you.

Improve your mood. A negative state of mind can affect your health, even increasing your risk of gum disease.

- Feelings of anxiety, loneliness, and depression create stress in your body, making it harder to fight off infection, like the kind behind gum disease.

- When you're down or tense, you may eat more sweets than normal or stop taking care of yourself in other ways. In one study, more than half the people said they neglected their brushing and flossing routine when they were stressed.

- Chronic stress means you've got more of the hormone cortisol circulating through your bloodstream, and that's been linked to a more damaging form of PD.

Do whatever it takes to feel better emotionally — talk to friends or a professional, exercise, get a good-night's sleep, or try other stress-busting therapies.

Flossing made easy

Wouldn't it be great if you actually liked flossing? If somehow it were less messy, less of a chore, more fun even.

Forget the fact that flossing can reduce your risk of gum and heart disease, whiten your smile, and give you better breath. Go have fun. And what could be more fun than a new gadget.

> Pop a piece of cinnamon gum and chew away the bacteria that cause bad breath. Cinnamic aldehyde, a natural compound in the bark of the cinnamon tree, is used to flavor gum, candy, and other food items. Researchers found it can kill up to 40 percent of the odor-producing bacteria in your mouth. Choose a sugar-free cinnamon gum like Dentyne Fire to freshen your breath without added calories.

- Flossers. These are, basically, a piece of dental floss on a handle. Some, called floss picks, have a point on one end for additional cleaning. Choose a style that fits comfortably in your hand and has a small enough head to fit in the back of your mouth. Some are completely disposable and others have heads you either toss or refill. These can cost as little as a couple of dollars, but they all need either refilling or replacing.

- Electric flossers. If you're going to buy one power tool for your bathroom, skip the electric toothbrush and buy this. Research shows they clean just as well as manually flossing, but since most people already brush regularly and don't floss, this is where your extra dollars should be spent. All the major manufacturers carry at least one model, starting at less than $10.

- Irrigation devices. These send a steady or pulsing stream of water through a nozzle you direct at the spaces between your teeth. A month-long study showed that using some kind of oral irrigation device was just as good at removing plaque and reducing gum bleeding and inflammation as flossing. This may be your most expensive option, but it has fewer replaceable parts.

Surprising link spells double trouble

There's a dangerous connection between diabetes and periodontal disease (PD). Either one puts you at risk of the other.

Diabetes increases your chance of infection — almost any infection, including the kind that can lead to gum disease. In fact, PD is so common in people with diabetes it is considered a normal complication.

In turn, someone suffering from PD is flooded with inflammation, making diabetes a real threat. One study showed more than 90 percent of those with PD met screening guidelines set by the American Diabetes Association.

> Gum disease is not only physically unhealthy, it's emotionally damaging, as well. If you've lost teeth or have sores in your mouth, you are not as willing to smile and interact socially with others.

Protect yourself on both fronts. Fight gum disease with all the tactics discussed in this chapter and read up on blood sugar control in the *Diabetes* chapter.

Hearing loss

problems hearing on the phone • misunderstanding
others • constantly turning the TV volume up
• trouble hearing against background noise

Listen up. You don't want to miss out on a thing. Not an interesting conversation, an important phone call, or a loved one's voice. Start taking care of your ears right now and don't become one of the 36 million American adults with some degree of hearing loss.

Hearing is a purely mechanical process in your body — no chemical reactions involved — and what amazing mechanics they are. Your ears are extremely sensitive organs, made up of delicate bones, tiny hairs, and bundles of nerves. Sound waves are funneled down the ear canal, striking your eardrum and causing it to vibrate. The vibrations travel through the bones of your middle ear and onto the hearing or auditory nerve in your inner ear. Here, the vibrations become nerve impulses that are sent to your brain where they are interpreted as sound.

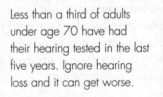

Less than a third of adults under age 70 have had their hearing tested in the last five years. Ignore hearing loss and it can get worse.

So what exactly goes wrong? Depends on the kind of hearing loss you experience.

- **Permanent.** Sensorineural hearing loss means there is irreversible damage to your inner ear or the auditory nerve. There are lots of potential causes including drug side effects, head trauma, and exposure to loud noise. Sometimes doctors cannot find a cause.

- Temporary. You experience conductive hearing loss when sound waves simply can't reach your inner ear. This may be due to fluid in your ear, a punctured eardrum, or a buildup of earwax. Your doctor can usually restore this kind of hearing loss.

- Gradual. Presbycusis is the type of hearing loss many people experience as they age. There are many causes including changes inside your ears, loud noise, head injury, illness, and circulation problems. This usually affects both ears equally and is such a gradual change most people don't realize they have a problem. Depending on the cause, this can be temporary or permanent.

Protect your ears to stay sharp. Losing your hearing is more than a minor inconvenience. It can impact your emotional and physical well-being.

- Memory. Hearing loss can subtly affect your memory and brainpower. Remembering new information takes up a chunk of your brain's resources. If those resources are being used instead to gather and interpret sounds, there's less effort put into memory. A study of older adults found those with mild or moderate hearing loss had more trouble remembering words read from a list than those with normal hearing.

- Balance. A recent study of over 400 women found those with hearing loss couldn't walk as fast as those without hearing problems and were twice as likely to have difficulty walking. By safeguarding your ears, you could improve your balance and cut your risk of a life-threatening fall.

- Stroke. Your risk of stroke is more than one and a half times greater if you've experienced a sudden hearing loss. See your doctor immediately, especially if you have heart problems.

- Safety. When voices or noises are muffled and indistinct, you may not clearly understand your doctor's advice or hear an alarm or warning.

- Socialization. It's embarrassing and frustrating when you can't join in conversations easily. You may begin to feel isolated or depressed. You can even come across as confused or uncooperative when the only problem is you simply can't hear.

Don't turn a deaf ear to hearing problems. Really pay attention to how you are interacting with others lately. Notice how often they must repeat questions, how many times you turn up the volume, and when you've missed out on vital information. Don't ignore warning signs you may be getting from friends and loved ones. This type of gradual hearing loss is something you should discuss with your doctor at your next checkup.

An otolaryngologist specializes in diseases of the head and neck, especially problems in your ears, nose, and throat. He is often called an ENT. An audiologist identifies and measures hearing loss. He cannot prescribe drugs or perform surgery but can help you choose a hearing aid.

On the other hand, if you wake up one morning with a plugged ear, don't panic. It could be something as simple as a head cold or too much earwax. Run through a couple of easy self-tests to get a fix on the problem.

- Hum a note. If it is louder in the blocked ear, you're probably suffering conductive hearing loss, which is temporary and usually reversible. Relax, wait a few days, and see if your hearing improves. If you hear the hum only in your other ear, it could mean you've got damage in your inner ear. Call your doctor.

- Talk to someone on the phone, switching the receiver from ear to ear. Determine if the hearing loss is equal in each ear or worse in one. Is sound only muffled or completely absent? Talk to your doctor about what you discover.

Depending on your type of hearing loss and its severity, your doctor may prescribe drugs like oral corticosteroids, a hearing aid, surgery, or special training. Don't resist this kind of assistance since it can open the world up to you again.

There are lots of easy things you can do now to keep your ears in tiptop condition.

5 tactics to fight hearing loss

Control use of pain relievers. Regular acetaminophen use, if you're under age 50, is almost guaranteed to cause hearing loss. Researchers followed almost 27,000 men for over 20 years and found those taking common over-the-counter (OTC) pain relievers more than twice a week showed changes inside their ears that affected how well they could hear.

Pain reliever taken more than twice a week	Increased risk of hearing loss		
	under 50 years old	50-59 years old	over 60 years old
aspirin	33%	33%	2%
other NSAIDs like ibuprofen and naproxen	61%	32%	16%
acetaminophen	99%	38%	16%

Unfortunately, these aren't the only medications that can damage your ears. According to the American Speech-Language-Hearing Association, there are about 200 prescription and OTC drugs that could cause temporary or permanent hearing loss.

- All aminoglycoside antibiotics are known to cause permanent hearing loss. Some names you may be familiar with are streptomycin, neomycin, and gentamicin.

- Vancomycin is another antibiotic that has been around for a long time. It has been more frequently prescribed in the last 20 years — and at higher doses than in the past — because of its use against a particularly nasty bacteria, methicillin-resistant *Staphylococcus aureus* (MRSA). Vancomycin can cause hearing loss especially in people over age 52.

- Loop diuretics for high blood pressure can trigger hearing loss or ringing in your ears. These side effects go away when you stop taking the drug.

- The most commonly prescribed form of hormone replacement therapy (HRT) is a combination of estrogen plus progestin, a synthetic form of the hormone progesterone. For years, scientists thought estrogen helped nerve cells and could protect a woman's hearing. They studied 124 postmenopausal women to see if this were true. To their surprise, estrogen was not protective. In fact, the women taking progestin experienced a 10 to 30 percent greater hearing loss than women taking estrogen alone or not taking HRT at all. The team of researchers plan to test whether or not this hearing loss is reversible.

Ask about the possible side effects of any medicine you plan to take. Never stop taking a prescription drug just because you think it might be affecting your ears or hearing. Talk to your doctor first.

Watch out for noise. You can hear because your inner ears contain small hair cells that convert sound vibrations into electrical signals. These signals travel to your brain where they are interpreted as sound. You only have a certain number of hair cells and when one is damaged or dies, you cannot grow a new one. Each hair cell you lose means your hearing is a little bit diminished.

Maybe someday scientists will learn how to grow new hair cells, but in the meantime, the most important thing you can do is protect the ones you have.

Noise is one of the major ways hair cells are damaged. It can be a sudden loud burst of sound or an ongoing exposure to noise above a certain level. According to the National Institutes of Health, 26 million Americans between 20 and 69 years old have permanent hearing loss due to loud noise. The good news — noise-induced hearing loss is 100 percent preventable.

> You can buy a batteries-included hearing aid on the Internet for about $10. But should you? Remember, no one is testing your hearing, fitting the device to you, or monitoring the fit for potential damage.

- Know what is loud. Any noise above 85 decibels can damage your inner ear. This includes motorcycles, gas lawnmowers, snow blowers, and firecrackers. For a more complete list of average decibel levels for everyday sounds, see the noise levels chart on the Internet at *www.asha.org/public/hearing/disorders/noise*.

- Shield your ears. Use earplugs or protective headphones whenever you're involved in a loud activity.

- Control the volume. Lower the maximum setting on your personal music player. Try talking at a normal conversation level while your headphones are on and music is playing. If you can't hear yourself clearly, your volume is too high.

- Choose in-ear-canal headphones. These allow you to keep the volume low on personal players even in noisy environments.

- Limit cell phone use. If the ear you normally use with your cell phone is unusually warm or feels full, you may be talking your way into trouble. A small study found those who had used a cell phone for more than four years and talked more than an hour every day were more likely to have high-frequency hearing loss.

Unplug the wax. Earwax serves an important purpose — it keeps dirt and debris from entering your ear canal. Too much also keeps sound waves from reaching your inner ear. Have your doctor take a look. If this is a problem, she can flush out your ears at her office and give you tips for keeping the wax under control.

Avoid ear infections. They aren't just for kids. As an adult, you can get an upper respiratory infection that settles in your ears. You may feel a temporary deafness because of the infection and swelling, but if it goes on too long, the damage can become permanent. Prevent getting a bug in the first place by washing your hands frequently, getting a flu shot every year, and seeing your doctor before an earache turns into something more serious.

Start your day with a supplement. Help your body by giving it more ammunition against the dangers of this noisy world.

- Folate. A brand new study showed that men over age 60 who had a high intake of the B vitamin folate from foods and supplements were 20 percent less likely to develop hearing loss. Folate's antioxidant properties may help protect your ear's delicate inner workings. Older research points out that folic acid supplements protected low-frequency hearing the most.

- Alpha lipoic acid (ALA) and coenzyme Q10 (CoQ10). Individually, these two supplements work hard to keep your body healthy. ALA helps convert sugar to energy and acts as an antioxidant to neutralize harmful chemicals known as free radicals. CoQ10 also turns sugar, as well as fat, into energy and is necessary to keep every cell in your body functioning normally. What's new and exciting is they protect against the cell damage and cell death behind age-related hearing loss.

- An antioxidant cocktail. A combination supplement containing magnesium, beta carotene — which the body converts into vitamin A, and vitamins C and E may prevent both temporary and permanent noise-related hearing damage if taken before you're exposed to loud noise. Several studies have tested this blend of nutrients anywhere from a month to a single hour before subjecting ears to loud sounds. In all cases, the individual elements weren't helpful, but the combination reduced hearing loss and cell death. Here's how much of each nutrient the U.S. Food and Drug Administration says is safe for adults.

Daily Tolerable Upper Intake Level	
vitamin A	3,000 micrograms
vitamin E	1,000 milligrams (mg)
vitamin C	2,000 mg
magnesium	350 mg

3 surprising hearing hazards

Life may not seem all that noisy, but you may be putting your ears at risk in some unexpected ways.

- A quiet day on the golf course could turn out to be a real ear-splitter. The new thin-faced titanium clubs produce quite a crack — some measuring in at 120 decibels. Keep ear plugs in your golf bag.

- Zooming down the open road with your convertible's top down sounds like a little slice of heaven — until you measure the roar of the wind and traffic. Experts say you'll cut some of the damage by rolling up your windows.

- Subway cars in New York City can save you gas but cost you your hearing. They were consistently above the safe noise level in public health studies. Passengers waiting on the platforms were most at risk. Wear in-ear-canal headphones with your personal music player at a low volume.

Hot trends in hearing technology

Bluetooth-enabled hearing aids. They work like a hearing aid plus a hands-free device, giving you access to cell phones, computers, and other electronics using wireless technology. Adapters let you hook into televisions and personal music players or upgrade a hearing aid you already have that didn't come with a built-in Blue-tooth receiver.

Implanted hearing system. A device, about one and a half inches around and one-fourth inch thick is surgically inserted into your skull just behind your ear. Wires beneath your skin connect it to sensors in your middle ear. Once the device is activated, it improves moderate to severe hearing loss from nerve cell damage.

> The FDA says do not use ear candles for any reason. They claim to draw impurities out of your ear canal, treating sinus infections, earaches, headaches, hearing loss, and even cancer. All you'll really get is a risk of burns and punctured eardrums.

Claiming to work better than a hearing aid, this system distinguishes between different kinds of sound, filtering out background noise. The pacemaker-type battery can last up to nine years. The Envoy Esteem device costs about $30,000 and is FDA-approved. For more information, visit *www.envoymedical.com.*

Speech recognition software. Soon you'll be able to add software called Clearcall to your digital hearing aid or cochlear implant. Research says it improves speech recognition by up to 50 percent.

Invisible hearing aid. Lyric is a revolutionary device that sits entirely within your ear canal and uses your outer ear to funnel sound directly into your ear. There's no surgery, and you can wear the

Lyric for months at a time. When the battery runs out, your doctor removes the entire device with a magnet and inserts a new one. It's sold on a subscription basis and includes new devices throughout the year. Learn more on the company's website, *www.lyrichearing.com.*

Unconventional treatments triumph over tinnitus

There may not be a cure for tinnitus yet, but there are certainly things you can do to relieve symptoms and improve quality of life. This ringing in your ears is usually caused by noise exposure and affects about 50 million Americans. Talk to your doctor about these treatment options.

Music therapy. German researchers took the favorite music of tinnitus sufferers and removed just the notes that matched the frequency of the ringing in their ears. After listening to this modified music for a year, the people said their tinnitus was not as loud.

Repetitive transcranial magnetic stimulation. Tinnitus may be caused by something going wrong in your central nervous system. This treatment uses a coil to create a magnetic field around your brain, which then generates an electric current to affect the overexcited neurons. In recent research, just five days of treatment significantly improved tinnitus symptoms for up to six months.

Acupuncture. A study out of Sao Paulo Federal University showed one session of acupuncture turned down the volume on tinnitus for a group of sufferers between the ages of 36 and 76.

Temporomandibular disorder (TMD) treatment. Sometimes two conditions are related. If you suffer from TMD, you have problems with your jaw, jaw joint, and the facial muscles surrounding the joint. After tinnitus sufferers were treated for their TMD, 83 percent said their tinnitus also improved considerably.

Hearing aids. Don't discount this long-established remedy. A recent survey found six out of 10 people suffering from tinnitus experienced minor to major relief when wearing hearing aids.

High blood pressure

often no outward symptoms • mini-stroke or TIA
• heart problems • kidney disease • vision problems
• stroke • dementia

One of the biggest threats to your brain is high blood pressure. This condition afflicts about 65 million Americans, making them 600 times more likely to develop dementia. If you want to keep your wits about you as you age, find out how to avoid this preventable and treatable condition.

Blood pressure refers to the force of your blood against the walls of your arteries. A blood pressure reading has two numbers. Systolic blood pressure, the top number, measures the force as your heart beats. Diastolic blood pressure, the bottom number, measures the force between beats.

The scary thing about high blood pressure is you can easily have it without knowing it. That's because it often comes with no symptoms at all. At least not until you suffer a transient ischemic attack (TIA), or mini-stroke, or develop heart, kidney, or vision problems. That's why it's important to get your blood pressure checked regularly.

High blood pressure can affect your brain in a few ways. It's the major risk factor for stroke, which is sometimes called a "brain attack." When you have a stroke, blood vessels become blocked or burst, cutting off blood flow to part of your brain and killing brain cells. Controlling your blood pressure is one way to shield yourself from stroke.

Several studies have linked high blood pressure to mental decline and memory problems. Because high blood pressure restricts oxygen to the brain, it also contributes to dementia.

Now researchers have found another possible explanation. High blood pressure may damage the tiny blood vessels that nourish your brain's white matter, the network of nerve fibers that lets your brain cells communicate. This leads to white matter lesions, a type of scarring linked to Alzheimer's disease and other forms of dementia. The higher your blood pressure and the longer it goes uncontrolled, the more white matter damage occurs.

You may eventually need medication — or a combination of medications — to control your high blood pressure. But lifestyle changes can also make a big difference. Try these surefire ways to get your blood pressure under control and keep your brain sharp for a lifetime.

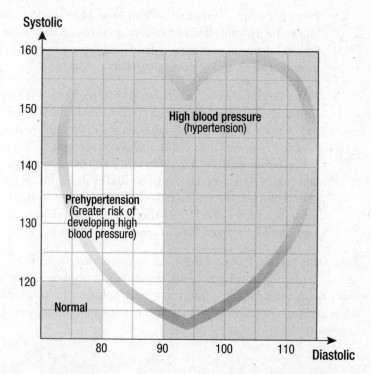

4 tactics to fight high blood pressure

Tweak your diet. Change how you eat, and you'll change your blood pressure numbers for the better. Take these three simple steps to gain control of high blood pressure.

- Slash sodium. Cutting back on sodium — to less than 2,300 milligrams a day — will help. Sodium causes your body to retain water, boosting your blood's volume. It also constricts small arteries, hampering blood flow. Both of these outcomes can raise your blood pressure. To make matters worse, a high-salt diet may even make blood pressure-lowering drugs less effective. Put away the salt-shaker and read food labels carefully to find low-sodium options. Beware of processed foods like cold cuts, canned foods, frozen dinners, salad dressings, snacks, and fast food.

- Boost potassium. This mineral helps lower blood pressure and blunts the harmful effects of sodium. Experts recommend at least 4.7 grams of potassium a day. Good sources include fresh fruits and vegetables, legumes, and dairy products.

- Add a DASH of good health. Sticking to the DASH (Dietary Approaches to Stop Hypertension) diet could take you the rest of the way. This plan emphasizes fruits, vegetables, and fat-free or low-fat dairy. It also includes whole grains, fish, poultry, and nuts, and it's low in lean red meat, sweets, and sugary beverages. Government studies show this eating plan is an effective way to reduce blood pressure. You can learn more about the DASH diet on the Internet at *www.dashdiet.org* and various government websites.

Shed some pounds. Losing weight can help you win the battle against high blood pressure. If you're overweight or obese, your body needs more blood — and this greater volume of blood means more pressure on your artery walls. Recent research found that for roughly every 2 pounds you lose, your blood pressure drops one point. Stay away from fad diets and other weight-loss gimmicks. The best and safest way to lose weight is to cut back on calories while increasing your physical activity.

Stay active. Regular exercise not only helps you lose weight, it also helps you lower your blood pressure. Being a couch potato, on the other hand, makes your arteries less elastic and harms their ability to dilate. You don't have to run a triathlon to reap the benefits of exercise. Gentle is effective. Simple things like walking, taking the stairs, and practicing tai chi can be enough to get your blood pressure numbers down. One review of more than 50 trials found that regular, moderate physical activity reduced blood pressure by an average of 4 mm Hg diastolic and 3 mm Hg systolic. Aim for 30 minutes of exercise each day.

> Timing is everything. If you experience side effects like leg swelling, headaches, or rash when taking the calcium channel blocker nifedipine, you may not have to switch medications — just the time of day you take it. A recent study found that taking the drug at bedtime — rather than in the morning — reduced side effects. Mention this study to your doctor if you are having side effects from this drug.

Reduce stress. When you're stressed, your body releases hormones that raise your blood pressure and speed up your heart rate. Chronic stress takes its toll on your arteries, leaving them stiff, rigid, and constricted. Learn how to cope with stress, and you'll do your heart — and brain — a favor.

Effective stress-relievers include exercise, relaxation techniques, and listening to music. Lightening your workload or personal schedule can also help. Working hard when you're fatigued can elevate your blood pressure.

Kick these habits to control your blood pressure

Now that you know what to do to keep your blood pressure under control, here's what not to do. Remember these six no-no's if you want to keep your mind sharp for life.

- Don't smoke. Chemicals in cigarettes constrict your blood vessels and boost blood pressure. If you're a smoker, quit this dangerous habit.

- Don't drink too much. Limit alcohol consumption to one or two drinks a day. Drinking more than that may raise your blood pressure.

- Don't stay angry. Anger constricts your blood vessels and reduces blood flow, but laughter has the opposite effect. Having a positive outlook may help keep your blood pressure in check.

> Here's some bitter news for grapefruit juice lovers. Grapefruit juice interacts with some blood pressure medications, such as calcium channel blockers. A substance in grapefruit juice blocks your liver's ability to break down these drugs, leaving you with dangerously high levels in your bloodstream. Ask your doctor or pharmacist about potential food-drug interactions.

- Don't isolate yourself. Loneliness may increase your risk of high blood pressure. Stay connected to friends, family, or community groups.

- Don't drink energy drinks. They may give you a boost of energy, but they also give you loads of caffeine, which can elevate your blood pressure.

- Don't indulge your sweet tooth. A recent study found that a high intake of fructose, found in soft drinks, baked goods, and candy, can raise your blood pressure.

High cholesterol

total cholesterol over 240 • LDL cholesterol over 160
• HDL cholesterol under 40 • triglycerides over 200

Mention high cholesterol and grown men start to cry. It's the death knell for drive-thru french fries and warm, gooey donuts. You wish, just once, there was something good to say about it — and now there is.

Cholesterol is a natural part of a healthy body. Although you get some from foods, you make about 75 percent of the cholesterol that's in your blood. And not all of it is bad. Among other things, it's used to produce cell membranes and some hormones. It's also the raw material for bile, which is important for healthy digestion. So why does cholesterol get such a bad rap?

It can't dissolve in your blood, so something has to take it to and from your cells. These carriers are called lipoproteins. One type, HDL or high-density lipoprotein, is considered "good" because it takes cholesterol away from your cells to your liver where it's passed from your body.

Eating foods high in saturated fat, trans fats, or cholesterol can increase your cholesterol levels. And that's not all. Some people inherit genes that cause them to make too much cholesterol. If you have a family history of high cholesterol, lifestyle changes might not be enough to lower it.

Another type of carrier is LDL or low-density lipoprotein, and it's considered "bad." It gives the cholesterol a ride to your body's tissues. If there's too much LDL circulating in your blood, it can slowly build up on the inner walls of the arteries that feed your heart and brain. Along with other substances, it forms plaque, a thick, hard deposit that clogs your arteries and makes them less flexible. This is known as atherosclerosis, and it means your heart has to work harder to pump blood through these stiff, narrow arteries. That means less nutrient- and oxygen-rich blood is able to circulate past this traffic jam. And if a clot forms and blocks the flow completely, you can suffer a heart attack or stroke.

This is bad news for your brain in two ways. When brain cells die due to a lack of oxygen or because of a clot-induced stroke, you can develop what's called vascular dementia. This is the second most common form of dementia after Alzheimer's disease (AD). In addition, according to surprising new research, strokes can trigger your brain to produce beta-amyloid protein, a key component of the plaques found in the brains of people who have AD.

	Total Cholesterol	LDL (bad) Cholesterol	HDL (good) Cholesterol
Dangerous	>240	>160	<40
Borderline	200-239	100-160	
Healthy	<200	<100	>60

A study of almost 10,000 people showed that those who had high cholesterol in their 40s — measured as more than 240 mg/dL — increased their risk of Alzheimer's disease later in life by 66 percent. More disturbing, if their levels were only borderline high, they increased their risk by 52 percent. Obviously, you want more HDL and less LDL cholesterol in your body to lower your risk of stroke. Read on to learn how you can lower your cholesterol.

6 tactics to fight high cholesterol

Treat yourself to soluble fiber. Add a few extra servings of fruit, beans, and cereal grains to your daily menu and you can lower your cholesterol. It's the soluble fiber in these foods that helps your body. It dissolves in your intestines, forming a gel that keeps cholesterol and fats from being absorbed into your bloodstream. As little as 3 grams of soluble fiber a day can drop your numbers, but if you bump it up to about 10 grams a day, you could see as much as a 5 percent drop in your LDL cholesterol.

Boycott bad fats. There are three cholesterol villains lurking in some common foods. Each of these will make your LDL levels rise.

- Saturated fat. You'll find this mostly in animal products like meat and dairy.

- Trans fat. This goes hand-in-hand with hydrogenated oils and fats. It's in a lot of fast foods, baked goods, and stick margarine.

- Dietary cholesterol. You don't have to swear off cholesterol-containing foods completely, but don't eat more than 300 milligrams a day. Watch out for egg yolks, shrimp, and whole milk dairy items like cheese, cream, and butter.

Focus on fabulous fats. Unsaturated fats are generally healthier for you than saturated fats. You may have heard of monounsaturated fat — olive oil and canola oil are good examples — and polyunsaturated fat — from safflower oil, corn oil, and fish containing omega-3 fatty acids. Be aware even healthy fats are high in calories, so eat them in moderation.

Let antioxidants fight your battles. Certain natural compounds in food stop free radicals from oxidizing low-density lipoprotein (LDL). That means the LDL cholesterol is less able to stick to your artery walls and form plaque. Flavonoids, especially, act as antioxidants in your body. You'll find them in a variety of fruits and vegetables, black tea, nuts, and seeds.

Get your heart pumping. According to experts, choosing all the right foods will only help your cholesterol if you also take part in some kind of regular, aerobic activity — something that gets your heart rate up. Not only will you raise your levels of good HDL cholesterol, you'll also lose weight. This is the most effective way to lower triglyceride levels, the form most fat takes when it is stored in your body.

Enhance control with enhanced foods. There's another group of foods that can help you naturally lower your cholesterol — those containing phytosterols. Also called plant sterols or stanols, you'll find them in fruits, vegetables, soybeans, breads, and peanuts. They help make up the structure of plant cell membranes. Plant sterols are also added to some food products, like margarines, mayonnaise, salad dressings, low-fat dairy, orange juice, chocolate, and meat. So how does eating what is essentially a plant cholesterol help lower your own cholesterol?

Lycopene is a perfect example of an antioxidant that keeps dangerous artery-clogging cholesterol from forming. Drinking just two glasses a day of lycopene-rich tomato juice increases LDL's resistance to oxidation.

The famous Nun Study, funded by the National Institute on Aging, followed 678 feisty members of the School Sisters of Notre Dame religious congregation, many of whom lived to be more than 100. Scientists discovered lycopene helped keep them active and independent.

Phytosterols interfere with your body's ability to produce and absorb LDL cholesterol. Both natural sources and foods enriched with phytosterol esters have been tested for how well they lower cholesterol. A major review of research found you can lower your LDL by around 9 percent if you stick to the recommended amount of 2 grams — or 2,000 milligrams (mg) — of phytosterols a day.

If you choose to add spreads and other enhanced foods to your diet, watch the calories and check the price. Here are some tasty and healthy natural sources.

Phytosterol content of selected foods		
Food	Serving	Phytosterols (mg)
Promise activ Light Spread	1 tablespoon	1,000
Benecol spread	1 tablespoon	850
sunflower seeds	1 ounce	150
corn oil	1 tablespoon	131
sesame oil	1 tablespoon	117
peanuts	1 ounce	62
pistachios	1 ounce	60
cashews	1 ounce	44
almonds	1 ounce	36
asparagus	8 medium spears	30
olive oil	1 tablespoon	30
margarine	1 teaspoon	12

Extra ammo to fight dementia

A class of cholesterol-lowering drugs called statins may also help protect your brain from Alzheimer's disease and other forms of dementia. In fact, one five-year study reported that statin users were about half as likely to develop dementia as those who didn't take the drug.

Although there's also been less than positive results from other research, some experts believe the type of statin you take may make a difference. Ask your doctor if you could benefit from statins.

> Even if you're thin, get your cholesterol checked regularly. People who don't usually gain weight are not as alert to how much saturated and trans fats they eat.

Hypothyroidism

sensitivity to cold • depression • fatigue • joint pain • muscle pain • dry skin • brittle nails • weight gain

A small gland you may never even think about produces one of your body's most critical hormones. It's responsible for how you use energy, it helps you stay warm, and it keeps your brain, heart, and muscles working properly.

The thyroid gland, part of your endocrine system, sits in the front of your neck, just below your voice box. One of the all-important hormones it produces is thyroxine or T4, which is carried via your blood to every cell in your body.

When you aren't getting enough thyroxine, many of your body processes start to slow down. You make less heat and energy. You feel colder. Your skin is dry. Your brain functions a little more slowly, and you become forgetful. An underactive thyroid, known as hypothyroidism, can cause a slew of mental symptoms, including slowed thought and speech, depression, and an inability to pay attention and focus. Some people call this "brain fog." Because of its impact on memory, perception, and judgment, experts consider thyroid hormones one of the major players in brain chemistry disorders. If hypothyroidism isn't treated, it can seriously affect your emotions and behavior.

Although you can develop hypothyroidism at any age, the older you are, the greater your risk. Women age 60 and older have the highest risk. It's very common for this condition to go undiagnosed. Part of the problem is symptoms of hypothyroidism are varied, can develop slowly over years, and can seem like a normal part of aging.

Many people associate their thyroid with iodine, and it's true there is a connection. Your thyroid has to have iodine to make thyroid hormones. But getting too little iodine is not a concern for most people — you get plenty from foods like seafood, chicken, beef, and pork. It's also added to baked goods, dairy products, and iodized salt. If you take any kind of seaweed supplement, you could be getting too much iodine — bad news for your thyroid. Getting too much iodine can cause or worsen hypothyroidism. Some weight loss supplements contain kelp, a kind of seaweed, so read package labels carefully. The recommended amount of iodine is 150 micrograms (mcg) a day. Most people get much more than that because of a high-salt diet. Experts recommend staying under 1,100 mcg of iodine a day.

A physical exam of your thyroid won't give you an accurate diagnosis. Ask your doctor for a simple blood test that measures thyroid-stimulating hormone.

4 tactics to fight hypothyroidism

Replace your missing hormones. There's no cure for hypothyroidism. But, by restoring the hormone your thyroid no longer makes, you can control it. Unless your case is severe, you're treated as an outpatient and simply take a pill every day for the rest of your life. Synthetic thyroxine is an exact match to the T4 your body would make if it could. It keeps a steady supply in your blood, so there are no highs or lows. The dose is determined

More than 30 million people in the United States suffer from a thyroid disorder. An additional 10 million are undiagnosed.

by your age and weight, the cause of your hypothyroidism, underlying conditions you may have, and any other medications you're taking.

Amp up your antioxidants. Ridha Arem, medical doctor and author of *The Thyroid Solution* , says certain antioxidants are vital for a healthy thyroid. They help it maintain an adequate supply of thyroid hormone, and they can clear toxic by-products out of your body. When your thyroid is out of balance, you don't have enough natural antioxidants in your body. Without them, free radicals run wild, overwhelming your cells, leading to deterioration and disease. The remedy for this is simple. Supplement your diet with plenty of vitamin C, vitamin E, and beta carotene, and you'll help keep your thyroid healthy and your mind clear. Good food choices are citrus, red peppers, leafy green vegetables, deep orange fruits and vegetables, and whole grains.

Take care of your heart. If your thyroid is underactive, you have a much higher risk of cardiovascular disease. Protect yourself by eating a heart-healthy diet and getting plenty of exercise.

Say goodbye to the blahs. Along with the brain fog of hypothyroidism, you can experience other symptoms like depression and fatigue. These keep you from thinking and feeling your best. To feel better, eat a healthy diet, drink enough water, exercise regularly, improve your sleep habits, and stay connected to friends and family.

Simple test saves your heart

Get your thyroid checked, especially if you are a woman over age 40. Even if you don't have symptoms of hypothyroidism, your heart may be in danger.

In a Norwegian study of more than 25,000 people, researchers observed that women with the least-active thyroids were 69 percent more likely to die from heart disease than women with normal thyroids. And this is just the latest in a long line of strong research.

Earlier research showed that women with only mild hypothyroidism were almost twice as likely as women without this condition to have blockages in their aorta. They were also twice as likely to have a history of heart attacks. A review of thousands of people with underactive thyroids without symptoms showed 65 percent had an increased risk of heart disease. New evidence suggests as your thyroid slows down, your blood pressure and cholesterol levels rise.

> There's a significant link between low thyroid levels and people who progress from mild dementia to Alzheimer's disease.

Inflammation fighters

salmon • sardines • walnuts • canola oil • olive oil • fruit • vegetables • whole grains • legumes • curry powder • ginger • garlic • cloves • dark chocolate

Inflammation is usually a good thing. The redness you see around a cut or the swelling you feel in your sinuses means your immune system is working hard to fight off bacteria or viruses. This kind of inflammation is called acute — it's typically severe, but it doesn't last very long. Once the danger has passed, your body shuts down this emergency response and things return to normal. You need acute inflammation to stay healthy.

Chronic inflammation, on the other hand, means your body's off switch isn't working. Your immune system continues in combat mode, churning out white blood cells meant to fight infection and chemicals designed to trigger further inflammation. It's a cycle that can go on for months, even years.

At first, you may not have any symptoms, but without a doubt, this nonstop, low-grade, silent inflammation is causing damage. It interferes with certain processes within your body and destroys tissues. Eventually, this damage puts you at risk of developing some very serious conditions, like diabetes, heart disease, Alzheimer's disease, arthritis, and even cancer.

Chronic infection often sets in motion the inflammation process. Do what you can to remove these surprising causes of infection from your life.

- stress
- obesity
- pollution
- viruses
- cigarette smoke

Although scientists cannot pinpoint exactly what causes this immune system malfunction, most agree you can fight it with a healthy diet, which includes a variety of foods and a controlled number of calories.

Eat to beat inflammation. Quell your body's destructive cycle with these tasty options.

- Cold-water fish contain a good supply of omega-3 fatty acids, which curb the amount of inflammatory chemicals you produce. In addition, your body takes an ingredient in fish oil and turns it into Resolvin D2, a substance that reduces inflammation. Good choices include salmon, sardines, and mackerel, but you can also get omega-3 fatty acids from walnuts and vegetable oils like canola, soybean, and flaxseed.

- Fruits and vegetables are jam-packed with antioxidants and other natural chemicals that battle the free radicals triggering damage at inflamed sites. Fill your plate with them generously and often.

- Whole grains and legumes give you a healthy dose of soluble fiber, the kind a new University of Illinois study says can change angry pro-inflammatory cells into healing, anti-inflammatory cells.

- Herbs and spices, like curry powder, ginger, garlic, and cloves, can certainly boost your inflammation-fighting diet. Add some zest to any dish while you fight an array of diseases.

- Dark chocolate is one treat you no longer have to deny yourself. Cocoa seeds contain plant chemicals that act as antioxidants to fight inflammation. Researchers found a small amount of dark chocolate can reduce levels of the inflammation marker C-reactive protein in your blood. The key here is moderation — no more than a small square two or three times a week.

Steer clear of troublemakers. The following choices bring something unhealthy and pro-inflammatory to the table. Some produce damaging free radicals, some routinely trigger allergic reactions, and some cause blood sugar levels to spike. All these things can lead to inflammation.

- trans fats from foods made with, or fried in, partially hydrogenated oils

- saturated fats in red meat and dairy foods

- processed foods

- refined carbohydrates, such as sugar and white bread

Easy test predicts heart disease risk

Inflammation is so thoroughly linked to illnesses like heart disease that your doctor may order a test for C-reactive protein (CRP) in your blood. Your body releases this substance in response to inflammation, so the higher your blood levels of CRP, the more inflammation present.

The American Heart Association and the Centers for Disease Control and Prevention say these CRP levels indicate your risk of heart disease:

below 1.0 mg/L	=	low risk
1.0-3.0 mg/L	=	average risk
above 3.0 mg/L	=	high risk

A CRP test is most useful if there are other indications that you have a moderate risk for suffering a heart attack or stroke. In that case, a high CRP level may prompt your doctor to take more aggressive measures to lower your risk, like prescribing medication to bring down your cholesterol or putting you on an aspirin regimen to reduce the chance of blood clots.

3 ways inflammation fighters keep you sharp

Save your heart from harm. It may be strange to think that your arteries can become inflamed. You certainly don't feel it like you would a sprained ankle — no tenderness or heat. But just the same, inflammation occurs deep inside your body.

It often starts with a small injury to the cells lining your arteries, perhaps due to an infection or exposure to a toxin, like cigarette smoke. This damage switches on your immune response, calling out the troops — white blood cells.

They mill around the area, directing your blood vessels to leak fluid into the surrounding tissue, causing swelling and the cell death that turns into scar tissue. Then some low-density lipoprotein (LDL) cholesterol floats by, snags on the damage, and begins to build up into plaques. These plaques get larger, partially blocking your arteries and making it harder for blood to flow through — just like a river gets dammed by floating debris.

Eventually, the plaques can get so numerous and so large they cut off blood flow and oxygen to your heart — and you experience pain known as angina. If things become completely bottlenecked, a blood clot forms. Clots can stay put and keep everything shut down or break free and travel to other places in your body causing even more trouble, like a stroke or heart attack.

This condition, known as atherosclerosis, develops after many years, but it began with a not-so-small thing called inflammation.

Boost brain defense. No one believed it at first. Experts thought the brain was pretty well protected from the damaging effects of immune system-induced inflammation — mostly by the blood brain barrier. This is a dense layer of cells separating your brain from the rest of your body and shielding it from potentially harmful substances, like hormones and toxins. Then three things were discovered that turned this theory around.

- Brain inflammation became one of the newest characteristics of Alzheimer's disease (AD).

- Common anti-inflammatory drugs were shown to sometimes protect against the development of AD.

- High blood levels of C-reactive protein (CRP), a natural marker of inflammation, indicated a greater risk of AD. In fact, it seemed to appear before any outward symptoms of AD or vascular dementia. Because CRP is actually poisonous to nerves and nerve tissue, it could be directly responsible for cell death in your hippocampus, the part of your brain responsible for forming new memories and storing old ones.

As brains age, they become more sensitive to inflammation and oxidative damage from free radicals. One solution is to give yourself some added ammunition through foods that quell inflammation and fight oxidation.

Derail diabetes. Inflammation triggers insulin resistance, which can lead to diabetes. This, in turn, creates further inflammation. It's a distressing cycle, but one you can break with a little know-how and a good plan. Here's the story.

Inflammation tells your body to produce increasing amounts of specific proteins that make you less responsive to insulin. In other words, your cells don't allow the insulin to move glucose inside. Your pancreas tries to fix this by producing even more insulin, but you just end up with a lot of insulin and glucose circulating through your bloodstream. This insulin resistance is a major risk factor for type 2 diabetes.

If you already have diabetes, your immune system is overly active and your immune cells churn out a higher-than-usual amount of inflammatory chemicals. This leads back to more proteins affecting insulin response.

In addition, once you're insulin-resistant and your pancreas no longer produces enough insulin to overcome the resistance, you face another issue. Insulin normally controls a particular protein, called FOXO1, which regulates other inflammatory chemicals that interfere with insulin signaling. Without enough insulin, FOXO1 can run wild, giving the go-ahead for a flood of even more inflammatory chemicals.

You've got to have the right amount of insulin and use it properly to control how much sugar or glucose is in your blood. Changing blood sugar levels affect your mental abilities by restricting how much glucose reaches your brain as fuel and by causing damage to the inside of your artery walls, setting you up for reduced blood flow.

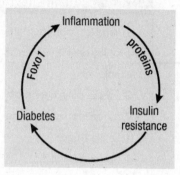

Perhaps the critical question is, which comes first, insulin resistance or inflammation? Right now, experts don't know. Your job is to adopt an anti-inflammatory diet and healthy lifestyle that will keep both inflammation and diabetes at bay.

Watch out for inflammation triggers

Let's say you bump your head. Hard. This kind of trauma may kill hundreds of thousands of neurons, or brain cells. That's not good, but it may not be devastating. Then your inflammatory response kicks in — a flood of killer cells swamps the injury site, portions of your brain tissue swell, and so on. This could potentially kill millions of neurons. And that is devastating.

This example shows how your body's response to injury — called secondary inflammation — and not the injury itself could be behind many chronic brain disorders. Protect yourself from physical trauma, like a head injury, and fight conditions, like atherosclerosis, that can set off silent inflammation.

Cabbage soup makes for a robust meal on a cold winter's day. Anti-inflammatory spices and vegetables make this meal a soothing delight.

Soothing slow-cooker cabbage soup

1 head of cabbage, torn into 2-inch pieces

1/2 lb. beef, chuck or shoulder, cut in small cubes

canola oil

2 10-oz. cans beef broth

1 12-oz. can carrot juice

1/2 tsp. sugar

1 tsp. cinnamon

1 tsp. ground cloves

1/2 tsp. ground ginger

1 cup carrots, sliced

1 cup celery, chopped

1 tsp. celery seed

1 cup onion, coarsely chopped

salt and pepper to taste

Braise beef cubes (you may substitute ham or sausage) in a skillet with a small amount of canola oil.

Place beef broth in a large slow-cooker and add carrot juice, sugar, cinnamon, ground cloves, ground ginger, carrots, celery, celery seed, chopped onions, and salt and pepper.

Add cabbage pieces and the braised meat and cook in your slow-cooker on the high setting for 3 hours, stirring occasionally.

Makes 4 to 6 servings

Insoluble fiber

whole-grain bread • whole-grain cereal • wheat bran
• brown rice • seeds • vegetables • fruit skins

Like a mysterious gunslinger in a Western, fiber is just passing through. After riding into town and saving the townspeople from the bad guys, the hero rides off into the sunset.

That's kind of how fiber works. Fiber, the part of plants your body can't digest or absorb, does not stick around in your body. It just does its job and moves on.

Fiber comes in two main varieties — soluble and insoluble. Soluble fiber can be dissolved in water, while insoluble fiber cannot. Many foods contain both types of fiber, but one may predominate. For example, oats and legumes are good sources of soluble fiber, while wheat bran and whole grains provide insoluble fiber. Both types of fiber protect your health, but they use different mechanisms of action.

1/2 cup wheat bran	11.3 g*
1/2 cup Fiber One cereal	11.1 g
1/3 cup All Bran cereal	7.2 g
1/2 cup kidney beans	5.9 g
1/2 cup frozen peas	3.0 g
1 cup of raspberries	2.4 g
1 tablespoon flaxseeds	2.2 g
1 slice of pumpernickel bread	1.5 g

* grams

Soluble fiber slows the emptying of your stomach to delay the absorption of some nutrients and lower LDL cholesterol. Learn more about the benefits and sources of soluble fiber in the *Soluble fiber* chapter.

Insoluble fiber adds bulk to your stool and speeds it through your intestines quickly to keep you regular and prevent constipation. It may also help control your weight and protect you from heart disease, stroke, diabetes, cancer, and diverticulosis.

Chances are you're not getting enough fiber in your diet. After age 50, men should aim for 30 grams of fiber a day and women should strive for 21 grams a day.

You can find insoluble fiber in whole-grain breads and breakfast cereals, brown rice, cauliflower, green beans, potatoes, broccoli, asparagus, carrots, zucchini, cucumbers, tomatoes, seeds, and fruit skins.

Eating more insoluble fiber doesn't just help your digestive system. It also has direct and indirect benefits for your brain.

5 ways insoluble fiber keeps you sharp

Improves your mood. You make decisions every day. Sometimes you use logic, carefully weighing the pros and cons before choosing. Other times, you just go with a gut feeling. These approaches may seem completely different, but recent research suggests that your gut and brain are closely linked.

While conventional wisdom says that psychological stress can cause physical problems, like irritable bowel syndrome (IBS), the reverse may actually be true. In other words, problems with your gut may affect your mental health.

That's because your gut and brain share some surprising similarities. Like your brain, your gut has a large network of neurons. Called the enteric nervous system, this network of

Motivated to add more fiber to your diet? Good idea. Just don't go overboard. Adding too much fiber too quickly can lead to unpleasant side effects, like gas, bloating, stomach cramps, and diarrhea. Introduce more fiber into your diet gradually. Make sure to drink enough fluids, too. Otherwise, the extra fiber can cause constipation.

neurons communicates with your brain and spinal cord. Both your brain and your gut depend on serotonin, the feel-good neurotransmitter that also plays a role in digestion and the perception of pain. In one study, people with IBS had significantly lower levels of serotonin in the lining of their guts.

Some drugs that lift your mood, like antidepressants, may also help with symptoms of digestive disorders, such as Crohn's disease or IBS — which includes diarrhea and constipation.

Constipation often goes hand in hand with a low mood. It may be both a symptom and a cause of depression. When you have smaller, less frequent bowel movements, the toxins in stool hang around longer and increase their chances of being reabsorbed by your body.

Boosting your intake of insoluble fiber — a tried and true cure for constipation — may also have a beneficial effect on your brain. One study found that people who ate high-fiber cereals had a more positive mood, as well as less emotional distress and fatigue than those who ate a low-fiber diet. They also had fewer mental difficulties.

Stymies stroke. Strokes happen when blood vessels in your brain become blocked (ischemic) or burst (hemorrhagic). Either way, the results can be devastating. Fortunately, insoluble fiber may provide some protection.

Studies suggest that a diet rich in fiber, particularly cereal fiber, lowers your risk of stroke. In one study, a 10-gram increase in fiber cut stroke risk by 41 percent in men with high blood pressure, while a 10-gram boost in cereal fiber slashed their risk by 67 percent. Another study found that women who ate the most cereal fiber had lower risks of both stroke, in general, and hemorrhagic stroke compared to those who ate the least.

Even if you do have a stroke, a high-fiber diet may cushion you from its damages. According to a recent study of 50 stroke victims, those who typically ate the most insoluble fiber had less-severe strokes and better chances of recovery. High blood pressure and obesity are both major risk factors for stroke, and previous studies have shown that people who eat a lot of insoluble fiber have lower blood pressure and lower body weight.

In one small study, people who ate insoluble fiber in the form of whole wheat and brown rice lowered both their systolic and diastolic blood pressures. The high-fiber, whole-grain diet also helped them control their weight.

Foils heart disease. While a stroke attacks your brain directly, heart disease represents an indirect — but still very serious — threat to your brain. Keeping your heart healthy helps keep your brain in tip-top shape.

Several studies have noted a link between insoluble fiber and lower risk of heart disease or heart failure. This has surprised some experts because soluble fiber is the kind that lowers cholesterol. While the mechanism remains unclear, insoluble fiber could help by lowering blood pressure and the risk of blood clots.

French researchers found that people who ate the most total and insoluble fiber improved several risk factors for heart disease, with lower blood pressure and lower levels of cholesterol, triglycerides, and homocysteine. They also were less likely to be overweight. To achieve these results, the researchers recommend getting at least 25 grams of fiber each day, while aiming for 30 to 35 grams for even more benefits.

Part of fiber's success could come from its anti-inflammatory powers. A recent University of Massachusetts study found that people who ate the most fiber had a 63 percent lower risk of having high levels of C-reactive protein (CRP), a marker of inflammation that indicates a future risk of heart disease and diabetes. For insoluble fiber, the benefit was even greater — a 75 percent reduction in the risk of high CRP.

Thwarts diabetes. Diabetes doesn't just affect your blood sugar. It can also affect your brain. Research indicates that eating more insoluble fiber may be an easy way to stop diabetes before it starts.

One study found that high cereal fiber consumption reduced the risk of developing diabetes by 28 percent, while an analysis of nine other studies determined it lowered diabetes risk by 33 percent. Exactly why insoluble fiber helps isn't clear, but there are some hints.

In a small German study, a boost in insoluble fiber improved insulin sensitivity by 13 percent in overweight or obese women. Researchers recommend eating more cereal, fruits, and vegetables rich in insoluble fiber as a way to reduce insulin resistance and lower your risk of diabetes.

Inflammation also plays a role in diabetes — and insoluble fiber may help squelch it. A British study found that older men who ate very little fiber or cereal fiber had a greater risk of developing diabetes. On the other hand, those who ate more fiber had lower levels of CRP and other markers of inflammation.

> Breathe easier with a bowl of cereal. A recent study found that fiber — and specifically cereal fiber — helped reduce the risk of developing chronic obstructive pulmonary disease (COPD), a group of lung disorders that includes chronic bronchitis and emphysema. Adding more whole grains to your diet may make things a whole lot easier for your lungs.

Controls weight. Extra pounds put you at extra risk for dementia. Being overweight also makes you more susceptible to heart disease, stroke, and diabetes. Think of insoluble fiber as a heavy-duty tool to help keep you slim.

In a Dutch study of more than 89,000 Europeans, a higher intake of fiber, especially cereal fiber, was linked to a slight reduction in body weight and waist size over a six-year period.

Canadian researchers demonstrated how insoluble fiber works — by making you feel fuller. Men who ate cereal that contained 33 grams of insoluble fiber had smaller appetites and ate less during their next meal than those who ate white bread or a low-fiber cereal. The high-fiber cereal also helped keep blood sugar levels under control.

In a similar study, those who ate high-fiber cereal — which had fewer calories than the low-fiber option — did not compensate by eating more at lunch. Because they filled up on insoluble fiber at breakfast, they ended up eating fewer overall calories. Eat more insoluble fiber to curb your appetite — and your risk of health problems.

Easy ways to boost your fiber intake

Fitting more fiber into your diet doesn't require too much effort. Just make some smart food choices and simple swaps.

- Start your day with a bowl of high-fiber cereal. Choose one with at least 5 grams of fiber per serving.

- Make sandwiches with whole-grain breads rather than white bread. Make sure bread has at least 2 grams of fiber per slice.

- Choose whole-wheat pasta over regular pasta.

- Opt for brown rice, barley, millet, bulgur, buckwheat, or quinoa instead of white rice.

- Eat the skin on your baked potato.

- Peel an orange instead of pouring some orange juice.

- Bite into an apple instead of spooning out some applesauce.

- Snack on popcorn or whole-wheat crackers instead of pretzels

- Enjoy bigger portions of vegetables, while cutting back on protein and starches.

- Swap beans and lentils for meat when possible.

You can also add supplemental fiber to most foods or drinks. In fact, manufacturers have been adding fiber to products like fruit juices, yogurts, and snack bars. But this type of fiber, called isolated fiber, may not provide the same health benefits of naturally fiber-rich foods. That's because you don't get any of the other nutrients — like vitamins, minerals, and phytonutrients — that make plant foods so good for you.

Whole-wheat pancakes

1 1/4 cup whole-wheat flour
1/4 cup wheat germ
1 1/2 tsp. baking powder
1/2 tsp. cinnamon
1/8 tsp. salt
1 1/2 cups skim milk
1/4 cup fat-free egg substitute
1 tbsp. unsalted butter, melted

Combine whole-wheat flour, wheat germ, baking powder, cinnamon, and salt.

Add skim milk, egg substitute, and melted butter.

Warm a skillet to medium-high heat and drop 1/4 cup of batter for each pancake. Don't crowd them. Cook for 2 minutes, flip, and cook for 1 more minute.

Raspberries in sauce

2 12-oz. packages frozen raspberries, thawed
1/3 cup sugar

Puree thawed berries in a blender or food processor and strain through a fine sieve to remove the seeds. Combine pureed raspberries with sugar and cook over low heat until well blended. Remove from heat and cool slightly. Serve warm or cold over pancakes.

Makes 2 servings

Surprising cause of brain inflammation

Some sources of fiber come with an added risk — gluten. A protein found in wheat, barley, rye, and oats, gluten poses a danger for people with celiac disease or a gluten allergy. It can cause cramps, diarrhea, or even severe intestinal damage. But gluten may also harm your brain. Gluten can spark brain inflammation and has been linked to dementia, nerve damage, anxiety, depression, and migraine headaches.

To test if you're sensitive to gluten, try eliminating it from your diet for a few months. This can be difficult, since it lurks in a variety of foods, including cereal, bread, crackers, pasta, soups, salad dressing, and beer. Then eat foods that contain gluten for several days in a row. If you notice an increase in fatigue, depression, or an inability to focus or concentrate, you may need to kick the gluten habit for good.

Iron

meat • fish • poultry • beans • cereals • fruit • leafy greens • nuts

Pumping iron doesn't have to mean a trip to the gym. It could mean pumping up your iron intake so you're more healthy and energized.

Iron helps make hemoglobin, which allows red blood cells to carry oxygen around your body. It makes brain chemicals like dopamine, norepinephrine, and serotonin and is required for various processes related to metabolism. Your body needs this essential mineral but doesn't produce it, so you must get enough in your diet. The iron in foods comes in two forms.

- Heme iron. This type, found in meat, fish, and poultry, is best for improving your body's iron levels.

- Nonheme iron. You absorb this kind of iron — which comes from plants — about half as well as you do heme iron. Get it from dried fruits, vegetables, grains, and nuts.

If you're over 50 years old, you need 8 milligrams (mg) of iron a day, unless you're a vegetarian. In that case, strive for more — about 14 mg a day — to make up for the absorption problems with plant sources. The average person gets about 10 to 20 mg of iron from their diet every day.

Don't overlook an iron overload. There are a couple of ways iron can build up in your blood and cause problems.

- Hemochromatosis. Suffer from this, the most common genetic disorder in the United States, and your body absorbs and stores too much iron — between five and 20 times more than you need. You may feel tired and achy or simply show high blood sugar levels or low thyroid function. Fortunately, this condition can be diagnosed early, thanks to genetic testing and simple blood work. An easy way to treat hemochromatosis — donate blood.

- Iron overdose. "Iron-poor blood" used to be a marketing catch phrase, prompting thousands of seniors to boost their blood with iron supplements. Today, you can get too much iron from multivitamins if you don't read labels carefully. According to experts, taking in more than 45 mg of iron a day can be unsafe.

3 oz. canned clams	23.77 mg*
1 cup General Mills Total Raisin Bran cereal	18 mg
1 cup canned pork and beans	8.20 mg
1 cup cooked lentils	6.59 mg
1 cup cooked spinach	6.43 mg
3 oz. pan-fried beef liver	5.24 mg
1 fast food hamburger	4.93 mg
1 cup canned prune juice	3.02 mg

* milligrams

Dodge the dangers of a deficiency. The World Health Organization says iron deficiency is the largest nutritional disorder in the world. For those with a few years under their belt, this is a real concern — a whopping 40 to 50 percent of seniors admitted to a hospital or living in a nursing home are iron-deficient. Here are some possible reasons why your iron levels could be low.

- Your diet may not include good sources of iron, especially if you eat lots of processed foods.

- Your ability to absorb nutrients decreases as you age.

- Any kind of chronic inflammatory disease like diabetes, heart disease, or rheumatoid arthritis, increases your risk of iron deficiency.

- Conditions that could cause internal bleeding, like ulcers, hemorrhoids, colon polyps, and gastrointestinal cancers, zap your iron stores.

- Your powers to absorb iron are impaired if you suffer from an intestinal disease or infection.

A blood test can determine if your iron is too low. Work with your doctor to correct the problem because without enough iron, you can develop a wide range of problems.

3 ways iron keeps you sharp

Fights the fatigue of anemia. Even a mild case of iron-deficiency anemia can leave you sluggish and feeling run-down. Don't ignore it. You're tired because you're not absorbing oxygen like you should. This can seriously damage your heart and reduce your ability to survive heart failure or a heart attack.

And you're weak because your muscles aren't fueled properly. You're less likely to exercise and more likely to fall. Other symptoms of anemia include:

- shortness of breath

- rapid heartbeat

- dizziness

- headache

- ringing in the ears

- irritability

- mental confusion

- loss of sex drive

> Men are at a higher risk for iron overload than women, perhaps because they eat more meat.

Although iron-deficiency anemia is just one kind of anemia, since it's based on a nutrient shortfall, it may be the simplest to understand and fix. Your doctor will test your blood's iron levels and talk to you about diet and supplements. If you're having trouble concentrating, don't let a simple deficiency in this trace mineral impair your mind.

Cracks down on memory loss. Several studies show iron-deficiency anemia increases your risk of dementia and can worsen existing dementia. Even if it's mild, anemia can sap your thinking.

Low iron in your blood could impact your brainpower in several ways. It can:

- reduce oxygen levels in your brain.

- make you more vulnerable to the damage from strokes or mini-strokes called TIAs.

- limit the amount of dopamine you produce, a brain chemical necessary for memory, learning, and attention.

- cause a decrease in thyroid hormones.

Perhaps the best argument linking iron to brainpower is that supplementing with iron seems to improve the thinking and learning problems in people with low iron levels.

> One study found Alzheimer's disease was twice as common in older people with anemia.

Just don't start taking extra iron on your own. Remember, you can develop serious health problems if you get too much of this mineral. Supplements may help only if you're deficient, so get your levels tested.

Relieves restless legs. A good night's sleep may seem out of reach if you suffer from the fidgety feeling of restless legs syndrome (RLS). This condition, characterized by an uncomfortable pulling sensation in your legs and the irresistible urge to move them, is thought to affect anywhere from 3 to 15 percent of the population. Iron deficiency appears to make RLS symptoms worse, while iron therapy can make you feel better.

The connection, again, is dopamine. Among its many jobs, this neurotransmitter is also responsible for triggering smooth muscle movement. Not enough iron means not enough dopamine.

Make the most of your iron

Adding iron to your diet is easy. Making sure the iron you eat is fully absorbed into your bloodstream is a little more tricky. Here are some tips to help.

- Don't take antacids or calcium supplements at the same time as your iron supplement.

- Take iron between meals with at least 8 ounces of fluid — not milk or caffeine-containing beverages.

- Drink a glass of orange juice. It's a healthy addition to any meal plus a good way to knock back your supplement. Vitamin C increases absorption of iron, especially nonheme iron.

- Pair meat or fish, sources of heme iron, with fruits, vegetables, and other sources of nonheme iron. This combination ensures you absorb the most nonheme iron possible.

- Team up with riboflavin. Liver and fortified cereals are not only great iron sources, but the riboflavin in them can boost your blood's response to the iron.

Simple steps to supplement safety

The amount of iron in multivitamins varies wildly. Know how many daily milligrams (mg) your doctor recommends and read labels carefully. For instance, one tablet of the multivitamin One-A-Day Women's contains 18 mg of iron. However, the Women's 50+ Advantage formula from One-A-Day contains no iron at all.

If your doctor has you taking a pure iron supplement, he may recommend ferrous iron, the more easily absorbed form. You'll probably see it labeled ferrous fumarate, ferrous sulfate, or ferrous gluconate. If these cause stomach upset, try chelated iron, time-release iron supplements, ferrous bisglycinate, or ferrous glycinate. They are slightly more expensive but less likely to cause an upset stomach.

Get your iron levels tested if you have diabetes because you're in danger of developing anemia. People who also suffer from chronic kidney disease or have damage to their large blood vessels, like in the heart, are at greatest risk. Correcting your iron levels can improve your quality of life.

L-carnitine

beef • lamb • poultry • fish • dairy

One little choice could peel back the years, giving you more energy than you can remember and fighting some of those invisible mischief-makers that hammer away at your youth and good health. That choice — carnitine.

Carnitine is a general term for an amino acid found in nearly all the cells of your body. You produce it naturally in your liver and kidneys, but you can also get it from foods and supplements. Slightly different forms include:

- L-carnitine. This is the only kind found in food. Although L-carnitine supplements are widely available and inexpensive, you absorb more of this nutrient from food sources.

- Acetyl-L-carnitine. Researchers use this form most often in studies of Alzheimer's disease and other brain disorders because it crosses easily into brain tissue.

- Propionyl-L-carnitine. This type seems particularly effective for heart disease and disorders affecting the blood vessels in your legs and feet.

So just what is all the fuss about? Basically, carnitine creates energy. It moves fatty acids into your cells' mitochondria, which are tiny power plants that burn fat and other nutrients to run practically everything in your body. Carnitine also:

- helps manufacture acetylcholine, an important neurotransmitter.

- transports toxic compounds out of your cells.

- helps move extra fuel from your cells into your blood-stream, where it's delivered to needier organs.

The Food and Nutrition Board of the National Academy of Sciences has not established a daily requirement of carnitine, so you won't find a DRI (Dietary Reference Intake) or RDA (Recommended Dietary Allowance) anywhere. If you eat an average diet that includes red meat and dairy, you probably get about 60 to 180 milligrams (mg) of carnitine every day. Relax. Even though that sounds like a lot, your body has a built-in safeguard to keep you from overdosing on carnitine. The excess is simply passed in your urine.

3.5 oz. lamb	190 mg*
3 oz. beef steak	82 mg
3 oz. ground beef	70 mg
3 oz. pork	24 mg
1 cup whole milk	8 mg
3 oz. cod	4 mg
1/2 cup ice cream	3 mg
2 oz. American or Cheddar cheese	2 mg

* milligrams

Is it enough? Yes. Consider that strict vegans — people who don't eat any animal or dairy products at all — get only about 10 to 12 mg of carnitine a day and are not considered deficient. This shows how efficient your body is at producing and storing carnitine. There are, however, instances where a carnitine deficiency could be an issue.

- You have a metabolic disorder where your body simply cannot make enough carnitine or use it properly.

- You're taking a medication that interferes with carnitine production.

- You are age 70 or older and no longer produce and store carnitine as you used to.

4 ways L-carnitine keeps you sharp

Helps heal a broken heart. Carnitine can really zero in on problems that stem from your heart. Here are three heart conditions you can tackle naturally with carnitine-rich foods and supplements.

- Intermittent claudication. When plaque builds up in your arteries, a condition called atherosclerosis, blood has a harder time flowing to all the distant parts of your body, especially your legs. Without enough blood, your muscles don't get the oxygen and nutrients they need to perform well. Even something as simple as walking can cause them to ache or cramp. This pain is called intermittent claudication. People who have it find it hard to walk even short distances at a slow speed. A number of studies have shown supplementing with about 2 grams of propionyl-L-carnitine a day helped those with intermittent claudication walk longer, faster, and with less pain. Experts believe carnitine improves how your leg muscles use energy.

- Angina. Chest pain is nothing to take lightly. In fact, you should never treat yourself. But if your doctor gives the go-ahead, try adding propionyl-L-carnitine to your conventional treatment. There's good evidence it can help some people with stable angina reduce their symptoms and even let them exercise without pain.

> Up to 86 percent of the carnitine you get from foods is absorbed in your small intestine and passed into your bloodstream.

- Heart attack. Your heart is one of the hardest-working muscles in your body. For that reason, large quantities of carnitine are concentrated here to ensure the cells make all the energy you need. When your heart is damaged — like after a heart attack — carnitine levels drop, leaving it weak and vulnerable. Several studies show if you take L-carnitine supplements soon after a heart attack, you cut your risk of suffering another one. In addition, you're less likely to experience chest pain and an irregular heartbeat, develop heart failure, or die of heart disease. It took 4 grams of L-carnitine a day and one year, but 80 people who had recently suffered a heart attack showed remarkable improvement.

Dulls the pain of diabetic neuropathy. The high blood sugar levels of diabetes can eventually damage the nerves in your arms, legs, and feet. This condition, called diabetic neuropathy, causes pain, numbness, tingling, and a burning sensation. Early studies suggest 2 to 3 grams of acetyl-L-carnitine a day can significantly improve these symptoms and even return normal feeling. Experts believe carnitine may provide extra energy to damaged nerve cells, helping them heal, and it may cue your brain to make more of a natural pain reliever.

Puts the brakes on dementia. There's no easy fix for dementia, but you can find hope in many places. And that's just what researchers have for acetyl-L-carnitine — hope. Admittedly, not all study results are positive, but many show a real benefit for people with early-onset Alzheimer's disease (AD) or those suffering from mild cases of this type of dementia. The theory is that this amino acid, by ramping up cellular energy production, can slow down the mental decline that is part of AD. The amounts of carnitine used in research varied from 1.5 to 3 grams a day.

Get your doctor's approval before taking this much, and while you're asking, find out about pairing acetyl-L-carnitine with an alpha-lipoic acid supplement. This combination gave better results than either compound alone.

Builds a better body. Want a little more spring in your step and little less weight on the scale? L-carnitine might help you reach that particular goal. It's been proven to boost muscle and reduce fat, plus relieve fatigue. You just may have more energy to exercise and feel better doing it.

Smart supplement strategies

Carnitine supplements may be the way to go if you need more of this amino acid than you can get from foods. Even though many supplements are available over-the-counter, talk to your doctor before you buy, and keep these things in mind.

- Don't substitute one form of carnitine for another.

- Avoid D-carnitine. This form competes with natural L-carnitine.

- High doses of acetyl-L-carnitine can make your urine, breath, and sweat have a fishy odor.

- Acetyl-L-carnitine can increase the effect of your blood-thinning medication.

- Don't take extra carnitine if your thyroid levels are low since it can make this problem worse.

> Good news for people with diabetes. Carnitine could boost the amount of fuel your cells burn, clearing extra sugar from your blood.

Magnesium

legumes • seeds • nuts • leafy green vegetables • whole grains • fish and shellfish

Just call it the smooth operator. Magnesium really knows how to make sure everything in your body runs smoothly and trouble-free. From keeping your nerves and muscles relaxed, to your blood circulating easily, this essential mineral is involved in hundreds of different chemical reactions. Magnesium helps you:

- break down carbohydrates, proteins, and fats.

- store energy in your muscle cells.

- keep a steady heart rhythm.

- regulate blood sugar levels.

- maintain a healthy immune system.

- preserve bone strength.

In fact, it's hard to find a system in your body that does not depend on magnesium to function properly.

Although you can't make your own magnesium, it's easy to get from many foods that should already be a part of your healthy diet. Basically, any food high in fiber is generally high in magnesium — like whole grains, beans, peas, seeds, and nuts.

Adult men should get 420 milligrams (mg) of magnesium a day, while women need 320 mg. Unfortunately, about 90 percent of Americans don't get as much of this important mineral as they should. Symptoms of a deficiency are wide-ranging. You could experience muscle weakness or spasms, a change in heart rate, headaches, high blood pressure, sleep problems, nausea, or depression.

5.6 oz. cooked halibut	170 mg*
1 oz. roasted pumpkin seeds	156 mg
1/2 cup trail mix	117.5 mg
1 cup cooked brown rice	84 mg
1/2 cup cooked spinach	78.5 mg
1 oz. almonds	76 mg
1/2 cup black beans	60 mg
3 oz. king crab	54 mg

* milligrams

Talk to your doctor to see if an underlying condition could be causing your magnesium shortfall. If you're older, he might recommend you take a supplement because you no longer absorb nutrients from food like you used to. Because not all multivitamins contain a full daily dose of magnesium, read labels carefully. You might need a separate magnesium supplement.

Experts say it's virtually impossible to get too much magnesium from food, but there is a danger of overdosing with supplements — don't get more than 350 mg from them in one day. Check the labels on any product you take regularly since laxatives, antacids, and calcium supplements often contain magnesium.

Healthy kidneys can usually get rid of extra magnesium quickly, but if you're getting a lot through supplements or if your kidneys aren't up to par, you could experience magnesium toxicity. The most common symptom is diarrhea.

6 ways magnesium keeps you sharp

Helps you dodge the dangers of diabetes. A peanut butter sandwich could protect you from type 2 diabetes. It all starts with a small but critical role magnesium plays in helping enzymes break down glucose — or blood sugar. Without this first step, you're well on your way to insulin resistance, which means your body produces insulin, but it's less effective in lowering blood sugar.

Just by bumping up your daily magnesium intake another 100 milligrams (mg) — the amount in two slices of whole-wheat bread and a couple of tablespoons of peanut butter — you could reduce your risk of diabetes by 15 percent. This benefit was most obvious in people who were magnesium-deficient or had the lowest intake of magnesium.

In addition, women who got close to the recommended daily amount cut their risk of developing metabolic syndrome by 38 percent. This collection of health problems includes high cholesterol, high blood pressure, and abdominal fat and puts you at greater risk of heart disease and diabetes.

Relieves the pressures of high blood pressure. Relax your muscles. Relax your arteries. In fact, just relax. Magnesium is here to rescue you from high blood pressure. It keeps your nerves from becoming overexcited and allows blood to flow easily through even the smallest arteries.

A recent South Korean study found that 300 mg of magnesium oxide a day for 12 weeks lowered blood pressure in people who suffered from high blood pressure but were otherwise healthy. If you're already taking medication to lower your blood pressure, talk to your doctor before supplementing, but you can safely make some magnesium-smart changes to your diet.

Says nuts to depression. Your neurons are damaged when you get too little magnesium, and your chances of suffering from the blues skyrocket. Eat more magnesium-rich foods like nuts, seeds, and whole grains, however, and you could lift yourself out of that funk. In fact, it's commonly reported that magnesium can turn around major depression in as little as a week.

Close to 6,000 people in Norway proved that simply boosting the amount of magnesium in their diet improved their mood. And a separate 2008 trial found supplementing with 450 mg of magne-sium every day was as effective as taking a daily 50 mg dose of the commonly prescribed antidepressant imipramine (Tofranil).

> Watch out for the most notorious side effect of magnesium — diarrhea. Almost all forms of the mineral can act as a laxative, although you're probably most familiar with magnesium hydroxide, better known as Milk of Magnesia. If you need a powerful laxative, look for a product containing magnesium sulfate. It's the most potent form. To tone down the effect your magnesium supplement may have on your intestines, take it with food.

Lets you catch 40 winks. Good sleep gives your brain and body time to recharge. You think better and faster, and you generally feel energized. Poor sleep, on the other hand, leaves you tired and sluggish.

Ever think a night of tossing and turning could be from a magnesium deficiency? Not enough of this important mineral can cause the electrical activity in your brain to change, leading to disturbed sleep. Magnesium may also help ease chronic low-grade inflammation, which has been linked to poor sleep. If you choose to supplement, try taking it just before bedtime to quiet overexcited nerves and help you fall asleep.

Saves your ears from harm. Loud noises cause microscopic damage in your ears that can have king-size consequences. In reaction to the assault, free radicals cause blood vessels to constrict inside your ears, restricting the flow of blood, oxygen, and other nutrients.

Natural and unprocessed foods are best when it comes to magnesium. Many great food sources are stripped of this valuable mineral when they're refined or cooked. For example, one slice of whole-wheat bread contains a whopping 23 milligrams (mg) of magnesium. A slice of white bread — only 6 mg. And when you boil spinach, you lose about one-third of its magnesium.

The result is something called noise-induced hearing loss (NIHL). Magnesium restores order mainly by relaxing your blood vessels but also by controlling glutamate, a brain chemical that sends information between nerves.

A combination of magnesium plus the vitamins A, C, and E is especially powerful in protecting against NIHL. Several studies have tested this blend of nutrients anywhere from a month to a single hour before subjecting ears to loud sounds. In all cases, the individual elements weren't helpful, but the combination reduced hearing loss.

Cracks down on memory loss. It's a fact. The older you get, the less magnesium you get — down to half the recommended daily amount. Does this deficiency have anything to do with age-related loss of memory and thinking skills? A groundbreaking animal study suggests it does.

More magnesium in the brains of both young and old rats improved several different types of learning and memory. During the trial, using standard supplements to get levels high enough to show benefits led to magnesium-induced diarrhea, so the researchers developed a special form of magnesium that loads directly into the brain. They found brain activity critical to learning and memory increased in those on this unique formula.

It's not commercially available yet, but this is certainly something to look for in the future. In the meantime, keep your magnesium levels high and your thinking skills sharp by including lots of magnesium-rich foods in your diet.

Soak up some magnesium and say 'ahh'

It all began on a little 17th century farm in England — a place called Epsom. When his cows refused to drink from his well, a farmer noticed the water tasted bitter. Further examination showed it also had amazing healing properties. The powdery substance distilled from this water was magnesium sulfate and became known as Epsom salt. The rest is history.

You may take a bath with Epsom salt to soothe scratches, a rash, or sore muscles. What you may not realize is you're also absorbing some magnesium through your skin, boosting your magnesium levels by as much as 35 per-cent. To get this kind of benefit, sprinkle three cups

> Hard water contains magnesium. Water softeners remove it.

of Epsom salt in your tub and soak for about 12 minutes, a couple of times a week.

Supplement secrets: become a savvy shopper

Two things determine how effective a magnesium supplement is.

Percentage of magnesium. Supplements are a combination of magnesium and another substance, usually salt, an amino acid, an organic acid, or a fatty acid. The actual amount of magnesium in a supplement is called elemental magnesium. Product labels should tell you how much elemental magnesium you'll get in each dose. When an independent lab tested several types, they found the elemental magnesium ranged from 75 milligrams (mg) a dose to 750 mg.

Bioavailability. This refers to how well your body absorbs the magnesium. Certain magnesium compounds are called chelated, and they are absorbed better than others. They include:

- magnesium glycinate
- magnesium stearate
- magnesium aspartate
- magnesium chloride
- magnesium taurate
- magnesium lactate
- magnesium citrate

Percent magnesium in supplements

Magnesium oxide	60%
Magnesium glycinate	50%
Magnesium carbonate	45%
Magnesium hydroxide	42%
Magnesium citrate	16%
Magnesium lactate	12%
Magnesium chloride	12%
Magnesium sulfate	10%
Magnesium gluconate	6%

Nonchelated forms — magnesium oxide, magnesium sulfate, and magnesium carbonate — are not absorbed as easily. In addition, any magnesium supplement that is enteric-coated means there is an outer layer on the tablet that keeps it from dissolving in your stomach. You don't absorb this type as well, either.

Medicine and your brain

drugs that keep you sharp • the placebo effect • pill taking tips • off-label uses • meds that cloud your mind

Medicine began with purely natural elements — things like willow bark, poppy, digitalis, and quinine. Many of these evolved into modern-day drugs, like aspirin and morphine. Scientists still rely heavily on nature for inspiration, but they design and create most medicines you take in laboratories.

> The Lord hath created medicines out of the earth: and he that is wise will not abhor them.
>
> *(Ecclesiasticus 38:4-5)*

Drugs can be harmful or helpful, but they all have one thing in common — they somehow change the way your body works, often by mimicking your natural chemicals or altering them in some way.

For instance, a pain reliever can keep injured cells from making and releasing a chemical called prostaglandin, which sends pain messages to your brain. Drugs for depression can act as a stimulant, triggering the release of adrenaline, making you feel more alert. Sleep aids can imitate the hormone melatonin, which prompts your body to slow down and go into sleep mode.

Whether or not a drug is good for you depends on many things including:

- how much you use.

- how often you use it.

- how quickly it gets into your bloodstream.

- what other drugs or foods you take with it.

- your body size and chemistry.

Where it all starts. The path any medication travels in your body is dictated by the kind of drug it is and what it is supposed to do.

- Swallow a pill or liquid medication and your stomach's digestive juices immediately start to break it down. From there, the active ingredients pass into your bloodstream and then they are off to other parts of your body.

- Sometimes digestive juices are too powerful for a drug and would essentially destroy it before it got a chance to do its job. Enteric-coated pills are covered with special ingredients that seal the medicine until it passes safely through your stomach and arrives in your small intestines. If you split or crush enteric-coated pills and capsules, you bypass this safety mechanism.

- Often a drug must act directly on a certain body part. That's when you might get an insulin shot, use an inhaled bronchodilator, or dab on a topical antibiotic ointment.

Protect your brain. No matter how you take medicine, all roads eventually lead to your brain. There, something called your blood brain barrier (BBB) plays a very important role. This dense layer of cells separates your brain from the rest of your body, protecting it from potentially harmful substances, like hormones and toxins, and allowing other materials, like nutrients, to cross through.

Keep your BBB as healthy as possible. These things can damage it to the point it can't stand guard the way it should:

- high blood pressure

- infection

- head trauma

- inflammation

Sometimes the BBB locks out helpful medications — those meant to act upon brain cells or fight brain diseases, like Alzheimer's. This is one problem scientists face on their quest for more effective drugs.

Placebo effect: when hope is the best medicine of all

Do you accept the power of positive thinking? Thousands of people unwittingly do it every day. It's called the placebo effect — when your medical condition improves following a therapy or treatment simply because you expect it to.

Perhaps your doctor sends you on your way with a prescription drug not really designed to help your condition. Or maybe you're eager to try vitamins or another alternative remedy. You start to feel better and the question arises, did the treatment work or did you simply believe yourself well?

Skeptics can't argue with the fact that sugar pills labeled as a stimulant have been proven to raise blood pressure and heart rate, and dummy sleeping pills can, in fact, make people drowsy.

Many experts attribute the placebo effect to the power of the mind. They say you, as a patient, can use emotions and thought processes to heal yourself.

The bottom line, choose a treatment you have confidence in and face all aspects of your healthcare with a positive attitude.

4 surprising ways medicine affects your brain

Hormone therapy helps you stay sharp. There's a critical window of opportunity when taking estrogen may help your brain hold on to memories. But wait even a few years to begin hormone replacement therapy (HRT) and the negatives outweigh the positives.

It's been quite the roller coaster of opinion over the past few years for women wanting a definite answer to the question, "Is HRT safe for me?" The latest research supports the idea that this amazing hormone can save your memory, but generally only for younger women — those in the years leading up to menopause and in early postmenopause. Estrogen seems to stimulate activity in the part of your brain used for working memory. Women several years past menopause not only won't help their memory, they'll be at increased risk of heart disease, stroke, and breast cancer if they take estrogen. There are still many issues you should discuss with your doctor, including which type of estrogen is best for you and how long you should take it.

> Think your memory is slipping? Don't go to the doctor first. Check the table in this chapter to see if you're taking any of the medications listed. Then go to your pharmacist and make sure she knows every prescription and over-the-counter medication you take. Discuss side effects and interactions with her. Then ask your doctor which medications you can safely change or eliminate.

Off-label use can repair stroke damage. A stroke means loss of oxygen to your brain, often with devastating consequences. However, prompt medical treatment can be a true lifesaver. For instance, the clot-busting drug t-PA works wonders after an ischemic stroke but only if given within the first four hours. Now there are treatments that may give stroke sufferers a little more time.

- A common antidepressant takes some of the urgency out of post-stroke treatment as it helps restore brain function. People who received escitalopram (Lexapro) within three months following a stroke scored higher on thinking, learning, and memory tests than those taking a placebo. Experts believe this type of antidepressant encourages the growth of nerves that may help mend damaged mental abilities.

- A substance commonly used to treat cancer may protect your brain from a stroke's devastation. Bryostatin 1 comes from a moss-like sea organism and, if given within the first 24 hours after a stroke, prevents cells from dying and encourages the growth of connections between nerves.

Doubling up means longer benefits. Standard drug treatment for Alzheimer's disease usually includes one of these drugs.

- Cholinesterase inhibitors (CI) slow the breakdown of acetylcholine, a chemical needed to form new memories. There are a handful on the market, including Aricept, Exelon, and Razadyne.

- Memantine (Namenda) is the only NMDA receptor antagonist approved by the FDA for Alzheimer's. It helps regulate levels of a specific brain chemical, glutamate, that's important in learning and memory.

Neither class of drug cures Alzheimer's. The most they can do is improve symptoms in some people, often for only several months.

The latest news is that many people are seeing remarkable results when they combine these two drugs. A Harvard study found that people with Alzheimer's treated with a cholinesterase inhibitor plus memantine cut the rate of mental decline in half, compared with those taking a CI alone. In addition, the longer they took this combination of drugs, the greater the benefits.

Familiar drugs can kill your memories. The most common cause of memory loss is not Alzheimer's disease — it's a negative reaction to prescription or over-the-counter medications. The good news is most memory loss, thinking problems, and physical reactions like dizziness, sleeping issues, or tremors, are reversible.

As you age, you become more sensitive to drugs, your body doesn't eliminate them as quickly, and you're more likely to take multiple medications. All that increases the likelihood you'll have a negative reaction to a drug. And because many seniors expect to develop memory or thinking problems with age, they don't suspect that new pill they're taking is the culprit.

The largest source of negative mental effects on seniors is a group of drugs having anticholinergic properties. This means they interfere with the chemical acetylcholine, which carries information between nerves. When acetylcholine isn't allowed to do its job, you experience memory and attention problems, confusion, and even hallucinations.

Hundreds of prescription and over-the-counter drugs act as anticholinergics, including sleep aids, antihistamines, antidepressants, and blood pressure medications. They don't fall into one single category. Experts believe up to half of all seniors take a drug with anticholinergic properties at least once a day.

So before you blame senility or Alzheimer's, talk to your doctor or pharmacist about every single medication you're taking and make sure you're not taking certain drugs. Remember, a feeble mind is not a natural part of getting older.

Should you say no to soy?

Soy foods contain nutrients very similar to the female hormone estrogen. These natural estrogens, or phytoestrogens, have spawned a controversy over whether or not soy helps or hurts your brain.

The latest review of all the research shows that people eating tofu, a soy food product, a couple of times a week had worse memories, while those taking soy supplements showed improvement in their mental abilities. Overall, half the studies reviewed were positive, half negative. Even though soy can fight cholesterol and cancer, the benefits as you age are not so black and white. That's why if you're over age 65, some experts say to stop eating this popular health food and avoid the possibility it can wreak havoc on your brain.

Medications that may cause memory loss, confusion, or hallucinations		
Drug category	Commonly prescribed for	Examples of brand names
analgesic combinations containing diphenhydramine	pain, sleep problems	Advil PM, Excedrin PM, Tylenol PM
cholinergic receptor blockers	bladder control	Ditropan, Detrol, Enablex, Vesicare, Sanctura
antihistamines and sedating antihistamines	colds, allergies, sleep problems	Benadryl, Sudafed, Sominex, Nytol
H2-antagonists	ulcers	Tagamet, Zantac, Pepcid
benzodiazepines	anxiety, sleep problems	Ativan, Xanax, Lunesta, Ambien, Sonata
opiates	pain	Vicodin, Percocet, Percodan, Fiorinal, Demerol
tricyclic antidepressants	depression, chronic pain	Limbitrol, Triavil, Asendin
fluoroquinolone antibiotics	infections	Cipro, Levaquin, Floxin, Flagyl

Simple tricks to remember your meds

Remembering to take your medication can sometimes be a life-and-death issue. Just as important is remembering that you've already taken it, since a double dose can be as dangerous as a missed dose.

The first step is to make a list of all your medications and when you're supposed to take each one. Discuss the list with a family member and ask for help — two brains are better than one. Then consider one or more of these tools that may make it easier to remember.

- Use a pill box. Simple ones come with a compartment for each day of the week. More sophisticated styles have additional morning, noon, and evening sections. There are even electronic ones that come with alarms.

- Ask if your drug comes in a foil pack so it's obvious how many pills have been punched out.

- Buy a watch with an alarm.

- If you use a computer most days, take advantage of a simple alert program.

- As you're taking a pill, pause and associate it with an image. For instance, you spy a beautiful bird out the window. Later, you may remember you saw it as you took your medicine.

- Always take your daily dose at the same time you perform a daily task, like when you brush your teeth or before you walk to the mailbox.

- Do something physical and unusual every time you take your medicine, like patting yourself on the head. It will help you remember you already took your pill.

And be aware, studies suggest seniors are more likely to forget their medication on days when they are busy.

Melatonin

tart cherries • bananas • sweet corn • tomatoes • beets • cucumbers • barley • rice • ginger • sunflower seeds • oats • flaxseed

There's more to melatonin than meets the eye. This hormone, produced in the pineal gland in your brain, controls your natural sleep-wake cycle, but that's certainly not the whole story. Here are three surprising facts about melatonin you probably didn't know.

It's in your gut. Although it was first discovered in the pineal gland, experts have since learned there's significantly more melatonin in your stomach and intestines than anywhere else in your body. After you eat, melatonin is released into your bloodstream. Foods high in tryptophan — red meat, dairy, nuts, seeds,

1 cup pitted Montmorency cherries	2,325 ng*
1 oz. roasted sunflower seeds	822.15 ng
1 cup cooked white rice	158 ng
1 medium banana	5.9 ng
1 small tomato	4.55 ng

* nanograms

bananas, soy, tuna, shellfish, and turkey — are specific triggers. Eating these foods is one way to get a boost of this hormone.

It's a potent antioxidant. Melatonin does more than influence your biological clock. It's involved in regulating several body functions — affecting your immune system and stress response. It also seems to be effective against breast cancer, colon cancer, and fibrocystic breast diseases. It can cross the blood brain barrier, a dense layer of cells and tissue that protects your brain. It can also enter every cell in your body where its antioxidant properties help fight free radicals at the source.

Melatonin can make nightmares more intense.

You need very little. There's only a small amount of naturally produced melatonin in your body — about as much as in one tart cherry. Normally, that's enough, but you can get more from foods and supplements. Most vegetables, fruits, nuts, and cereals contain some, but in small amounts.

Supplements are available over the counter and are chemically identical to the melatonin your body makes. Just remember, melatonin is not regulated by the Food and Drug Administration, different brands may contain varying amounts, and different manufacturers may not agree on how much to take.

No one is sure how much added melatonin a person should get, but it seems to be safe. In one study, people taking high doses — 30 or even 60 milligrams a day — didn't suffer any harmful side effects. However you take it, melatonin is easily absorbed into your blood and all your tissues, and any additional melatonin you get amps up your power to fight free radical damage.

> Your brain may house your primary circadian clock, but almost every cell in your body has its own type of clock ticking away inside. These respond to various stimuli — such as food or exercise.

4 ways melatonin keeps you sharp

Restores sleep rhythm naturally. Quick, name five creatures that only come out at night. If your melatonin levels are where they should be, you didn't include yourself. Most people naturally cycle through periods of sleep and wakefulness that correspond to the hours of darkness and light. This cycle is regulated in part by your internal clock, which responds to signals from hormones like melatonin.

Let's travel through your day and see exactly what's happening.

- The sun comes up. When light hits your eyelids, you stop producing melatonin. You won't generate any more for about 12 hours.

- Gradually, your body warms up, it starts cranking out stimulating hormones like cortisol and testosterone, and your blood pressure rises. You begin to feel alert.

- Throughout the day, you really get in gear. Your coordination, strength, and reaction time peak after noon.

- Early evening, things start to wind down. Your body responds to the increasing darkness, and about 9:00 p.m., you begin producing melatonin. You start to feel sleepy.

- Sometime after midnight, you reach your point of deepest sleep and lowest body temperature.

- A new day dawns and everything starts over.

As you age, you make less melatonin and, as a result, may have trouble falling or staying asleep. That's when boosting your melatonin becomes a good idea. Eating foods containing melatonin or taking supplements at the right time of day — an hour or two before bedtime — can improve the quality of your sleep without making you feel drowsy the next morning.

You'll want to check out supplement labels before you buy melatonin. This is one case where more is not better. Massachusetts Institute of Technology (MIT) researchers found a standard dose of about 3 milligrams (mg) overloads the melatonin receptors in your brain to the point they stop working. One-tenth of that amount — or just 0.3 mg — is enough to help you fall asleep and maintain better quality sleep.

> Read supplement labels carefully to see exactly how much melatonin you're getting. You may see only its chemical name, either N-acetyl-5-methoxytryptamine or 5-methoxy-tryptamine.

If jet lag is your problem, follow these guidelines to restore a normal sleep pattern.

- Take melatonin one hour before you want to fall asleep on the plane, or take it at your destination between 10:00 p.m. and midnight.

- Continue taking melatonin for three or more evenings in a row after you arrive at your destination.

- The benefit is greater the more time zones you cross.

- There's less benefit if you're traveling west.

Melatonin helps you experience good, restful sleep, which means a sharper brain and higher energy levels.

Turns back the clock on aging. The very act of living and breathing causes microscopic damage inside your body. Oxygen interacts with your cells and produces harmful molecules called free radicals. These tamper with cells, tissues, and organs in ways that lead to many diseases and general aging. Anything that fights this oxidative stress keeps you healthier longer. As an antioxidant, melatonin does just that.

- It works against free radicals directly but also boosts the power of other antioxidants.

- It could help delay inflammation-related illnesses by neutralizing the inflammation caused by free radical damage.

- If given early enough, melatonin supplements can prevent your body from forming beta-amyloid proteins, a hallmark of Alzheimer's disease.

Brightens up seasonal depression. You might suffer from a certain type of depression if your biological clock is out of whack. Known as SAD, seasonal affective disorder usually hits people who are night owls — they sleep late, stay up late, have more energy late in the day, and are down in the dumps.

If this describes you and your depression is worse in the fall and winter, melatonin could help reset your body clock. But don't start popping supplements on your own. Timing is very important. Work with your doctor on a program that involves a sleep schedule, planned exposure to light, and low-dose melatonin supplements.

> Hormones are chemical messengers that act like spark plugs for your body, triggering various systems to action. Without them you couldn't grow, reproduce, digest food, or experience emotions.

Drops nighttime blood pressure. Your blood pressure goes through a daily cycle just like your sleep stages. It rises rapidly in the early morning hours, peaks in the early afternoon, then declines until it hits its low about 2:00 a.m. Experts believe this cycle is somehow connected to melatonin, since your blood pressure naturally drops just when the melatonin levels in your body are rising at night.

Taking additional melatonin at bedtime can make your blood pressure drop even more, without affecting your daytime blood pressure or your heart rate. This is good. Nighttime blood pressure that is significantly lower than daytime blood pressure protects your heart from damage.

For some people, there is no nightly decline in blood pressure — It stays high even during sleep. Melatonin supplements could be especially helpful for them.

> Melatonin could spell relief for tinnitus sufferers. Those who took 3 milligrams of melatonin a day for a month found their symptoms — continual ringing, hissing, or buzzing noises — improved and they had better quality sleep. Those with a history of the worst sleep showed the greatest improvement.

A study out of Boston found giving 2.5 mg of melatonin at bedtime to men with untreated high blood pressure improved their day-night cycle, causing their blood pressure to drop to more normal levels during the night.

High blood pressure is a serious matter, so don't take melatonin without discussing it with your doctor first.

Shop wisely for best sleep solution

You can buy melatonin supplements as regular tablets or capsules, or in special time-release formulas. Quick-release forms may work best if you need help falling asleep. Extended-release products give you a smaller dose of melatonin over several hours, perhaps helping you stay asleep throughout the night. And you no longer have to split pills yourself to get the smaller doses used in many sleep studies.

Melatonin may be good for your heart in several ways. As an antioxidant, it protects against heart attack and stops bad LDL cholesterol from sticking to your artery walls.

Monounsaturated fats

nuts • olives • vegetable oils
• seeds • fish • avocados

The world preaches low-fat. Spend any time in the grocery store or in front of the television and you're bound to think anything with the word "fat" in it must be bad for you. Not true.

You need some fat in your diet. It gives you energy and helps your cells grow. Fats make sure you can absorb certain nutrients and produce important hormones. Unfortunately, most people eat too much of the wrong kind of fat. There are basically two categories of fat — saturated and unsaturated.

- Saturated fat, which generally comes from meat and dairy, is considered a bad fat since it's the main dietary cause of high cholesterol and is linked to several diseases. Eating lean meats and low-fat dairy will help limit this type of fat.

- Unsaturated fats, including polyunsaturated fatty acids (PUFAs) and monounsaturated fatty acids (MUFAs), come from plant and marine sources and are actually good for you.

The majority of people don't understand the distinction between fats. A recent American Heart Association survey found that 80 percent of Americans didn't know unsaturated fat is an important part of a healthy diet.

That said, fat is still fat. Every gram of fat, regardless of the kind, contains nine calories. Eating too much of it, even the healthy unsaturated variety, can put on the pounds. Experts agree — the amount of fat you eat should not make up more than 25 to 35 percent of your total daily calories. Let's say you plan on getting 30 percent of your daily calories from fat.

Here's a quick rundown of the maximum total fat grams you should get in a day based on several calorie intakes. Keep in mind, most of these fat grams should come from MUFAs and PUFAs, instead of saturated fats.

If you eat this many calories a day	Don't eat more than this many total fat grams
1,200	40 g
1,500	50 g
1,800	60 g
2,000	67 g
2,200	73 g
2,500	83 g

3 ways monounsaturated fats keep you sharp

Control your cholesterol. It's official. There's so much solid evidence that olive oil, a primary source of monounsaturated fatty acid (MUFA), is good for your heart that even the government is convinced. The FDA is now allowing olive oil manufacturers to claim that eating about two tablespoons of this delicious oil every day may reduce the risk of heart disease.

Of course, to get this benefit, you must use olive oil instead of foods high in saturated fat, like butter. That's the kicker — replacing bad fats with good ones. In fact, substituting saturated fats with monounsaturated fats lowers your risk of heart disease more than replacing them with carbohydrates, especially if you have diabetes.

To keep your brain in tiptop condition, you need a strong heart and healthy, flexible arteries. This ensures a steady flow of oxygen and nutrient-rich blood. A high-MUFA diet does this primarily by reducing cholesterol.

10-12 macadamia nuts	16.8 g*
20 pecan halves	11.6 g
3 oz. pickled herring	10.2 g
1 tablespoon olive oil	9.8 g
1 tablespoon canola oil	8.9 g
5.5 oz. cooked salmon fillet	8.2 g
1 tablespoon tub margarine	5.2 g

* grams

"Bad" LDL cholesterol only sticks to your artery walls after it's been damaged by certain molecules called free radicals. Once attached to your arteries, it builds up and forms dangerous plaques. By protecting LDL from free radicals, olive oil short circuits this process. When people with high cholesterol completely removed saturated fat from their diets and replaced it with olive oil:

- their total cholesterol levels dropped an average of 13.4 percent and their LDL cholesterol levels dropped by 18 percent.

- they cut their risk of heart disease almost in half.

Other sources of monounsaturated fat are just as good for you. Eating about 2 1/2 ounces of nuts a day can lower cholesterol, as well. Fortunately, people with higher LDL levels showed the most benefit.

In addition to battling high cholesterol, olive oil and other MUFA-rich foods fight the over 7 million deaths caused by high blood pressure by keeping the walls of your blood vessels relaxed and dilated.

Preserve and protect your memory. The important Italian Longitudinal Study on Aging may have been the first to focus science's eye on the relationship between monounsaturated fats and dementia. Because fatty acids help keep the outer layer of brain neurons in good working order, this early research suggested they may also preserve brainpower. As you age, your brain requires more unsaturated fatty acids to get the job done, so experts proposed a MUFA-rich diet to keep healthy seniors sharp.

Since then, numerous studies have shown eating good fats is associated with stronger mental performance. Research following close to 7,000 seniors found that those who used olive oil for cooking and on the dinner table hung onto their memory and verbal skills longer than those who didn't. Who would have thought simply switching to an olive oil salad dressing could shield your brain from memory loss.

Fight the battle of the bulge. Cutting every bit of fat out of your diet is not necessarily the best way to lose weight. Monounsaturated fats can actually help you drop pounds. One type of MUFA called oleic acid causes a chemical reaction that stops your belly from feeling hungry. It triggers your small intestine to churn out the hunger-fighting compound OEA. This trips the switch that tells your digestive tract it's full. The result — less hunger for longer periods of time, which can help stop snack cravings.

> Olive oil and nuts, both major sources of monounsaturated fat, are an essential part of the Mediterranean diet. For more information about this healthy eating plan, see the *Age-related macular degeneration* and *Omega-3 fatty acids* chapters.

An Australian study compared a diet high in saturated fatty acids (SFA) — full of milk, butter, cream, cheese, and fatty meat — to one rich in MUFAs — olive oil, nuts, and avocados. Both groups ate the same percentage of total fat. It was just divided differently between saturated, monounsaturated, and polyunsaturated fats.

- All the people in the study said they felt full regardless of the type of diet they were on.

- Those on the MUFA diet felt more energetic than those on the SFA diet.

- The group eating foods high in saturated fat gained weight and fat, while those eating monounsaturated fats lost both weight and fat.

> One tablespoon of peanut butter, chunky or smooth, has less than 4 grams of monoun-saturated fat, while 1 ounce of roasted peanuts — about 28 nuts — has around 7 grams.

- Cholesterol levels rose in the SFA group and dropped in the MUFA group.

Make this kind of dietary change and you can also avoid dangerous belly fat — associated with an increased risk of heart disease and type 2 diabetes.

For this much butter or margarine	Substitute this much olive oil
1 teaspoon	3/4 teaspoon
1 tablespoon	2 1/4 teaspoons
2 tablespoons	1 1/2 tablespoons
1/4 cup	3 tablespoons
1/3 cup	1/4 cup
1/2 cup	1/4 cup + 2 tablespoons
2/3 cup	1/2 cup
3/4 cup	1/2 cup + 1 tablespoon
1 cup	3/4 cup

Bad news about a popular oil

There's a dangerous oil lurking in many popular foods that attacks your brain tissue, destroying clear thinking and memory. Called trans fatty acids, there's nothing we love — or hate — more.

Created during a manufacturing process that adds hydrogen to liquid vegetable oils, trans fats make commercially baked products taste good and feel appetizing in your mouth. They also allow oil for deep-frying to be used many times. That's why cakes, pastries, crackers, french fries, and various restaurant items are especially chock-full of trans fats. They do taste oh-so-good, but they are oh-so-bad.

Trans fats raise your harmful LDL cholesterol levels and lower your good HDL cholesterol. Eating them increases your risk of heart disease and stroke and is linked with a higher risk of developing type 2 diabetes.

But when it comes to your brain, trans fatty acids are sneaky little rascals. They worm their way into brain cell membranes and the protective covering around neurons. Once there, they interfere with the neurons' ability to communicate. That means neurons die and your brain can't perform as it should.

The danger to your health is so well established that some cities have banned the use of trans fats in their restaurants. As of 2006, the Food and Drug Administration (FDA) requires food manufacturers to list the amount of trans fats on the Nutrition Facts label.

The American Heart Association recommends restricting the amount of trans

> Olive oil is more than just a healthy helping of monoun-saturated fatty acids. Depending on where the olives are grown and when they are harvested, 8 to 10 percent of the oil could be made of polyunsaturated fatty acids. And with every spoonful, you're also getting a good dose of natural antioxidants.

fats you eat to less than 1 percent of your total daily calories. For instance, if you get 2,000 calories a day, take in less than 2 grams of trans fatty acids.

Unsaturated fats are liquid at room temperature, whereas saturated fats are usually solid.

A bit of good news — olive oil in its natural state does not contain any trans fatty acids.

Type of olive oil	How it's made	How it tastes	Best use
extra virgin olive oil	The highest quality oil made from ripe olives that are pressed immediately after harvest. No chemicals or high heat are used during the extraction process.	An intense taste and aroma with a fruity flavor	Use to season or drizzle on prepared food. Best used uncooked to appreciate its flavor.
virgin olive oil	Also made from the first pressing of the olives without chemicals or high heat.	Good flavor but slightly lower quality than extra virgin	Good for cooking or dressing food.
olive oil	A blend of refined and virgin olive oils, Sometimes described as "pure."	Mild flavor with just a hint of fruitiness	An excellent all-purpose cooking oil.
refined olive oil	Made by treating virgin olive oils with chemicals or heat.	Flavorless and odorless	Used in foods labeled "packed in olive oil."

5 things you should know about olive oil

- Buy olive oil in opaque or dark-tinted containers, since it can become rancid if exposed to heat and light. If you purchase a glass bottle, pick one from the back of the shelf that's been away from direct light. At home, store your oil in a cool, dark cupboard.

- You can refrigerate olive oil. It will become cloudy and slightly thick, but once at room temperature, it will return to normal.

- Olive oil stands up well to frying temperatures. Its smoking point, the temperature where it begins to break down and form trans fatty acids and other harmful compounds, is high — 410 degrees Fahrenheit.

> Omega-3 fatty acids, like those found in cold-water fish, are perhaps the most well-known type of polyunsaturated fatty acid. Nuts, seeds, and vegetable oils are other good sources of PUFAs.

- As it heats, it increases in volume, so less is required for cooking and frying.

- Olive oil forms a crust on foods as they fry that keeps the oil from penetrating into the food. That means foods fried in olive oil have a lower fat content than foods fried in other oils.

Music therapy

brightens mood • sharpens memory • improves movement • relieves stress • lowers blood pressure • eases pain • aids stroke recovery

Doctors are prescribing a natural remedy for Alzheimer's, Parkinson's, stroke, and depression. And it's not a drug, but something you'll enjoy every day. If that sounds like music to your ears, that's because it is. Music therapy may be just what the doctor ordered for a healthy brain and body.

Music therapy can take place with or without a professional music therapist and may involve listening to music, singing, or playing an instrument. Settings for music therapy include hospitals, rehab facilities, senior centers, and nursing homes. But simply listening to your favorite music in the comfort of your own home can also have a favorable effect on your brain and your health.

Experts do not know for sure why music helps — but evidence suggests that the areas of the brain involved in music also deal with things like language, hearing perception, attention, memory, and motor control. Music may help activate these areas and improve interaction between them.

Music may even help you avoid certain conditions in the first place. In the Bronx Aging Study, which followed 469 men and women older than 75 years of age for an average of five years, playing a musical instrument and dancing were among the leisure activities associated with a reduced risk of dementia.

As beneficial as music therapy can be, keep in mind that it should not be a substitute for conventional treatment. Serious conditions may still require the help of your doctor, medication, and other professional care.

But music can be a helpful addition to your treatment — and your life. Find out why experts have been singing the praises of music therapy.

5 ways music keeps you sharp

Assists with Alzheimer's. Even when you can't remember names, you may still be able to name that tune. Music, especially familiar songs, can help slow the progression of Alzheimer's disease.

Listening to music can help people with Alzheimer's reconnect with their memories and rediscover their personality. It can even help them recall names, faces, and words, according to a study by the Institute for Music and Neurologic Function in New York. If you have dementia, familiar tunes can help you relate to others and experience joy.

That's because music is powerful. Unlike verbal memory, music memory does not rest in one specific part of your brain. Since it's processed across many parts, it's harder to erase music from your mind. Not just any music will do. Songs that were popular when you were a teen or young adult have the most impact.

Actually making music also helps. According to the British Alzheimer's Society, singing familiar songs and learning new ones can help build self-esteem and ease loneliness for people with dementia. It may even delay the onset of memory problems. One study found that moving to music, playing rhythm instruments, and singing led to more group involvement and less disruptive behavior among people with dementia in nursing facilities.

Other studies have shown that music therapy can help retrieve seemingly lost memories and even help restore other cognitive functions, like reasoning, perception, and judgment. In one recent study, people with Alzheimer's remembered new verbal information better when it was sung and set to music.

Move to the beat to maximize your workout. A Japanese study found that music can help ward off fatigue during exercise. Another study found that specific rock and pop music can improve exercise endurance by 15 percent. Choose upbeat music, ideally with 120 to 140 beats a minute, for a moderate to intense workout.

Singing in a group, such as a church choir or community chorale, also provides beneficial social ties. People with more social ties are less likely to develop mental decline.

Provides help for Parkinson's. People with Parkinson's disease experience tremors, stooped posture, slow movement, poor balance, and a shuffling walk. Except when they hit the dance floor. Canadian researchers have found that dancing can provide temporary relief from the effects of the disease. Even listening to music and thinking about your dance steps can help. For best results, choose music you like that triggers fond memories.

While all kinds of dancing helps, one specific dance may provide extra benefits. A recent Washington University study found that tango lessons improved mobility and balance in people with Parkinson's. Lessons included stretching, balancing exercises, tango-style walking, footwork patterns, and dance with and without a partner. Movements specific to the tango — including turning, moving at different speeds, and walking backward — may be especially helpful. The social aspect of dancing also plays a role.

Brightens your mood. If you have the blues, try listening to the blues. Or to rock, pop, R&B, country, jazz, classical, or any other music you like. Music therapy can help fight depression and anxiety.

According to a Cleveland Clinic study, listening to music can ease depression symptoms by 25 percent. People in the study listened to either their favorite music or soothing music featuring piano, jazz, orchestra, harp, and synthesizer. A South Korean study found that music can improve depression, anxiety, and relationships in people with mental illness.

In a French study, New Age music reduced the levels of the stress hormone cortisol. Other studies found that music reduces stress and anxiety before and during medical procedures. Choosing your own music may provide the most benefit.

Simply relaxing while listening to soft, soothing music worked just as well as a massage for reducing anxiety in a recent study, leading researchers to suggest this approach as a cheaper alternative.

Aids stroke recovery. After stroke strikes, strike back with music therapy. Music can help with several aspects of stroke rehabilitation.

For instance, singing can help you learn to talk again. An area in the left side of your brain affects speech, but the right side of your brain processes language, melodies, and rhythms.

So while you may have trouble thinking of the right word or forming sentences, you may still be able to sing the lyrics to familiar songs. A technique called melodic intonation therapy helps you sing sentences set to music. Then you try to remove the melody, leaving you with a normal speaking pattern.

Music may also help restore your vision. One common side effect of stroke, called visual neglect, hampers your ability to track objects in either your left or right field of vision. A recent British study found that listening to pleasant music can help improve this defect. However, unpleasant music and silence do not. Researchers suspect the positive emotional response from pleasant music — which is really any music you like — improves signalling in the brain. Listening to music regularly also improves cognition and mood after a stroke.

Lullabies aren't just for babies. Studies suggest soothing music can help older people get a good night's sleep. You can buy compact discs specially designed to promote sleep, but any music you find relaxing should do the trick. Soft, slow music at bedtime may be a cheap, effective remedy for insomnia.

Tames high blood pressure. Music may even help you avoid a stroke in the first place. That's because it may lower blood pressure and improve blood flow.

In a recent Italian study, people with mild high blood pressure listened to classical, Celtic, or Indian music for 30 minutes each day while breathing slowly. Their systolic blood pressure, the top number in a blood pressure reading, dropped by an average of 3.2 points after one week and 4.4 points after a month. Combining relaxing music and slow, gentle breathing with a long, relaxed exhale just may help get your blood pressure under control.

A Temple University review of 23 studies found that music helps people with heart disease relax and may even lower their blood pressure and heart rate. Choosing your own music provides the most benefit.

Music you find joyful may have a beneficial effect on your blood vessels. In one small study, listening to joyful music widened blood vessels by 26 percent. On the other hand, listening to music that causes anxiety can narrow arteries by 6 percent.

> Pump up the volume at your own peril. Loud music can damage your hearing. In some extreme cases, it may even trigger a collapsed lung. Keep your iPod or MP3 player set at a safe volume. For more information, see the *Hearing loss* chapter.

But a recent Italian study suggests that, whether you like the music or not, your body automatically responds to it. Crescendos, or gradual volume increases, lead to narrowing of blood vessels and increased blood pressure and heart rate, while diminuendos, or gradual volume decreases, usher in relaxation, which slows heart rate and lowers blood pressure. Music that alternates between fast and slow tempos, like operatic music, could be best for your circulation and heart.

Go online for great music

These days you may have trouble finding a local record or CD store. But you don't have to leave your house to find new music. Just log on to the Internet to access a treasure trove of tunes.

Internet radio works by streaming audio, which works best if you have a DSL or cable connection. You can find a huge selection of music styles on the Internet, with many stations playing only the type of music you really like. Most stations don't interrupt your music with commercials. And, because it's free, you can't beat the price.

Seek out your favorite Internet station at *www.radio-locator.com*. Click on the pull-down menu beneath "find Internet streaming radio," and select the type of music you like. Then click on "go." Whether it's jazz or classical, news or nostalgia, you'll get a list of stations you can listen to for free.

Some stations let you design a custom music selection that fits your taste, offering selections based on songs you like. Give it a try at Pandora (*www.pandora.com*), Slacker (*www.slacker.com*), or Yahoo! Music (*new.music.yahoo.com*).

You can also buy individual songs online for less than a dollar. Instead of a physical record, tape, or CD, you get a digital music file you can play on your computer, copy to a CD to play in your car's stereo, or move to your MP3 player. Browse these popular websites that offer large lists of songs.

- iTunes *www.apple.com/itunes*

- Napster *www.napster.com*

- eMusic *www.emusic.com*

- Rhapsody *www.rhapsody.com*

- Classical.com *www.classical.com*

Paint a rosier outlook with art therapy

Music isn't the only art form that has scientific support. Art therapy, an established treatment for mental health since the 1930s, employs a wide range of creative outlets.

Art therapy can include drawing, painting, clay, or sculpture, as well as discussion and interpretation of art. Like music therapy, it can be done individually or in a group setting. Used in the treatment of anxiety, depression, and other mental and emotional problems, art therapy provides several benefits. It may lift your mood, improve self-esteem, and stimulate your neurological pathways. It also reduces stress and helps you relax.

Studies suggest that art therapy improves the quality of life of older people, including those with Alzheimer's disease. Participating in art therapy may make you happier and calmer. You may also lower your blood pressure and experience less dizziness, fatigue, and pain. Simply gazing at paintings you like may reduce pain, according to an Italian study.

So get in touch with your inner Renaissance man, and discover the healing powers of art.

Niacin

yeast • meat • fish • poultry • milk • eggs
• green vegetables • cereal grains • legumes
• seeds • peanut butter

These days, 3-D movies are all the rage. But when it comes to blockbuster health benefits, vitamin B3 has its own eye-popping effects.

Niacin, also known as vitamin B3, serves several functions in your body. It helps break down blood sugar for energy and acts as a vasodilator to widen your blood vessels and improve blood flow. Niacin also builds DNA and helps keep your digestive system, nerves, skin, eyes, and hair healthy.

If you don't get enough of this important vitamin, you may put your health at risk. A niacin deficiency leads to a condition called pellagra, which features itchy, inflamed skin, stomach pain, diarrhea, depression, headache, thinning hair, and dementia.

Fortunately, you can find niacin in many everyday foods, including meat, fish, poultry, legumes, and fortified cereals. Your body also converts dietary tryptophan — found in red meat, poultry, eggs, and dairy products — into niacin.

The recommended dietary allowance (RDA) for niacin is 14 milligrams (mg) for women and 16 mg for men. While you can easily get this amount through your diet, you may

1 cup Product 19 cereal	20.01 mg*
3/4 cup Total Raisin Bran cereal	19.99 mg
3 oz. beef liver	14.85 mg
1/2 chicken breast	14.73 mg
1 cup tuna salad	13.73 mg
1/2 halibut fillet	11.33 mg
1/2 roasted duck	11.27 mg
1/2 salmon fillet	10.34 mg

* milligrams

need higher doses for certain health benefits. That's where niacin supplements come in. Prescribed mostly to raise good HDL cholesterol levels, niacin can also give your brain and overall health a boost. Find out how this B vitamin can be A-OK for your brain.

3 ways niacin keeps you sharp

Fights Alzheimer's. Give your memory a boost with vitamin B3. Studies suggest that niacin can help prevent Alzheimer's disease and mental decline.

A recent University of California, Irvine study found that nicotinamide, the biologically active form of niacin, helped mice with dementia. In fact, demented mice that were given nicotinamide in their drinking water performed memory tasks as if they'd never had the disease. It even improved short-term spatial memory in normal mice.

Nicotinamide may work by lowering the levels of a protein that contributes to the tangles found in the brains of people with Alzheimer's disease.

Promising evidence also comes from an earlier study of older Chicago residents. In the study, people who got more niacin into their diet had a lower risk of developing Alzheimer's disease. They also had a slower annual rate of mental decline.

Because one study dealt with mice and the other involved participants who filled out a questionnaire to let researchers know what they ate, more research is needed before niacin can be recommended. But it can't hurt to add some tasty niacin-rich foods to your diet in the meantime.

Improves cholesterol levels. This is niacin's claim to fame and the reason most people take niacin supplements. High cholesterol contributes to heart disease, heart attacks, and stroke and even puts you at greater risk for Alzheimer's disease.

But not all cholesterol is bad. Unlike the artery-clogging LDL cholesterol, HDL cholesterol whisks cholesterol from your bloodstream to your liver and out of your body. As your HDL goes up, your risk of heart disease goes down.

That's where niacin comes in. Niacin helps mainly by raising levels of HDL cholesterol. In fact, large doses of niacin are the most effective way to elevate your HDL. They can boost HDL cholesterol by 15-35 percent. But that's not all niacin does. Niacin can:

- lower triglycerides by 20-30 percent

- reduce LDL cholesterol by 10-20 percent

Combined with a statin, niacin helps even more. According to a recent University of Washington study, the combination of a statin and niacin reduces heart attack risk by up to 90 percent.

In another recent study, niacin worked better than the cholesterol-lowering drug Zetia to slow the buildup of plaque in artery walls.

People in the study were already taking statins to lower LDL cholesterol. Those who took niacin also raised their HDL levels by more than 18 percent, while also significantly lowering their LDL and triglyceride levels.

Raising HDL cholesterol not only protects your heart — it also safeguards your brain. Dutch researchers studying more than 500 people who were 85 years old found that those with low levels of HDL cholesterol were more than twice as likely to develop dementia as the people with the highest HDL levels. The risk was four times greater when researchers excluded those with a history of heart disease or stroke. Researchers suspect that HDL cholesterol fights dementia by preventing the buildup of beta-amyloid or reducing brain inflammation.

Niacin already has multiple benefits. Now researchers speculate it may even help fight multiple sclerosis. In a study of mice, nicotinamide — a form of vitamin B3 closely related to niacin — helped prevent the degeneration of nerve fibers and reduced inflammation. More research is needed, but this promising treatment could be a cheaper, safer alternative to commonly used drugs.

Helps with stroke recovery. A stroke can be devastating — but niacin may help put you on the road to recovery. Researchers at Henry Ford Hospital in Detroit have found that niacin helps restore brain function in rats who had a stroke.

Niacin sparked beneficial changes in rats' brains, including the growth of new blood vessels and the sprouting of nerve cells. As one researcher put it, "niacin essentially rewires the brain." The HDL-boosting powers of niacin may contribute to its success, but other factors likely play a role, too.

Studies are in the works to find out if niacin also helps humans. If those results are as promising as the preliminary animal studies, niacin could be a cheap, safe, and easy treatment for people who have suffered a stroke.

Get tough on cholesterol

You'd have to eat like a king — or several gluttonous kings — to get enough niacin through your diet to improve your cholesterol levels. But niacin supplements can provide the right amount to do the job.

Niacin is available by prescription in regular and extended-release form, which is called Niaspan. Typical daily dosages range from 2-6 grams for niacin and 1-2 grams for Niaspan. A niacin-plus-lovastatin combination pill is also on the market.

You can also find several over-the-counter options, including niacin derivatives such as inositol hexaniacinate or inositol hexanicotinate, which contains 85 percent niacin. These types are often preferred by natural practitioners.

Whatever form you choose, do not take supplemental niacin without consulting your doctor.

> Here's some sunny news — vitamin B3 may help protect you from skin cancer. The sun's ultraviolet rays suppress your skin's immune system, leaving it more susceptible to cancer. A recent Australian study found that nicotinamide supplements counteracted this effect of UV radiation. That's not the only way nicotinamide helps your skin. Also known as niacinamide, it's a common ingredient in skin creams.

'B' aware of vitamin's side effects

Even though niacin is a natural vitamin found in a wide variety of foods, it can pose some serious problems if taken at high doses.

The most common side effect is flushing of your face and shoulders, which can occur at doses over 50 milligrams a day. You may experience reddening of your skin, burning, tingling, itching, and pain. Headache and stomach problems are other common issues, while some people report heart disturbances and temporarily lower blood pressure.

At high doses, niacin can contribute to gout, ulcers, diabetes, and liver damage. It may also boost your levels of homocysteine, a substance linked to heart attack and stroke.

Remember, these side effects only occur with supplemental niacin — which you should take only with a doctor's supervision. Niacin-rich foods will not put your health at risk.

If you do take niacin, you can take several precautions to reduce flushing. Start with a lower dose of niacin and gradually increase it. Slow-release formulations of niacin also help. Taking aspirin or non-steroidal anti-inflammatory drugs (NSAIDs) may lessen flushing.

You may also want to avoid drinking hot beverages or alcohol. Taking niacin with food not only counteracts flushing, but it also helps prevent upset stomach and ulcers.

Obesity

BMI over 30 • waist measurement over 35 inches for women and 40 inches for men

You're on your way to the gym to work off those extra pounds, but you can't find your car keys. Did you ever think you can't find your keys because you're overweight? Ridiculous.

The truth is, if you're a woman carrying too many pounds, you're twice as likely to have any type of dementia, including Alzheimer's disease, as a woman of normal weight. If you carry that weight mostly around your middle, you've almost tripled the likelihood you'll develop dementia.

There are several possible explanations for how body fat — and especially belly fat — affects your memory. Perhaps the most straightforward involves the often deadly triangle of obesity, heart disease, and diabetes. This triad spells trouble for healthy blood flow and affects how you're able to think in so many ways. Because excess weight is tangled up with blood pressure, cholesterol, and blood sugar, it's almost impossible to fix any of them without first controlling the amount of fat in your body.

Here are some other ideas that help explain the connection between weight and brain function.

C-reactive protein. There's an interesting link between inflammation, body fat, and dementia that may center around a specific protein called C-reactive protein (CRP). Your liver produces CRP after an injury, infection, or inflammation. It disappears when the injury heals or the infection or inflammation goes away. You generally don't have this protein if you're healthy.

If your CRP levels remain high for too long, experts think your risk of heart disease, stroke, high blood pressure, diabetes, and insulin resistance go up. Every body is different, but if you are overweight, you're more likely to have higher CRP levels. And CRP is associated with thinking and memory problems, as well as dementia.

A recent German study suggests if you're overweight, cutting calories may boost memory and brainpower by reducing inflammation and

> Before you start a weight loss program, see your doctor. She'll take a complete medical history to determine if you have any underlying medical conditions that could affect your goal. You'll also discuss family history, medications, and possibly your mental health.

improving your blood sugar and insulin levels. The people in the study with the largest weight loss also showed the biggest improvements in memory.

Leptin. Your fat cells produce this hormone to control hunger, possibly by signaling your brain when there is fat on your body. If you can't make leptin, your brain thinks there is no fat and trips your "hungry switch." You eat more and more in an attempt to get the leptin signal that fat is present. In some way, extra fat cells — and the amount of leptin — affect your brain function. Research published in the *Journal of the American Medical Association* says people with the lowest levels of leptin were about four times more likely to develop Alzheimer's disease than those with higher levels.

It's an easy, but life-threatening, journey from visceral fat — the kind that lies deep within your abdomen — to higher insulin levels to type 2 diabetes to dementia. If you stop this train at the first station, you may avoid a nasty destination.

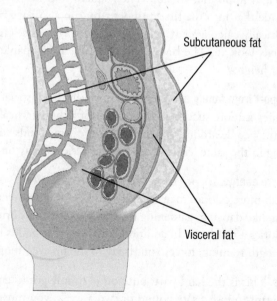

Subcutaneous fat

Visceral fat

5 tactics to fight obesity

Set reasonable goals. A sure way to fail in your quest for weight loss is to set the bar impossibly high. Determine what is a safe and realistic weight goal for you. You can have this discussion with your doctor, or you can use a standard calculation called the BMI (body mass index). This figures a measurement of your weight as it relates to your height. It doesn't measure body fat directly, but experts believe it is a good indication. These guidelines are from the National Institutes of Health:

- overweight — a BMI of 25 to 29.9

- obese — a BMI of 30 or greater

- extreme obesity — a BMI of 40 or greater

To find out where you stand now, calculate your BMI. Multiply your weight in pounds by 703. Then square your height in inches and divide that into the first number. You can also have your BMI automatically calculated at *www.nhlbisupport.com/bmi*. From this Web page, look at "The BMI Tables" to find a reasonable weight for your height.

Get support from family and friends. It's proven that a social support group means more success in the pursuit of a thinner, healthier you. When the people around you are eating the same foods you are and engaging in the same leisure activities, it's easier to stay on track.

Burn more energy. It's not rocket science. To lose weight, you've got to use up more calories than you take in. By doing something active and fun, like dancing, gardening, or walking, you can burn an extra 150 calories a half hour. In addition, anything that builds muscle, like strength training, forces your body to use up even more calories.

Eat less. This is the hard part, but you've simply got to cut calories. If you want to lose a safe pound or two a week, you must drop

500 to 1,000 calories a day. That can be hard if you rely on dieting alone. But combining a good eating plan with some exercise means you can lose more than by either strategy alone.

For example, set this goal — eat 250 fewer calories a day and burn 250 more calories a day. That gets you to your target of 500 fewer calories without extreme measures.

A super smart way to scale down on calories is with portion control. The American dining experience is loaded with heaping helpings and super-size options. Read about true serving sizes on food labels and really look at the amount of food on your plate. Extra calories are hiding in every spoonful.

Science proves cutting calories works for your brain. German researchers found that a group of overweight women who cut their daily calories by 30 percent lost an average of 5 pounds and improved verbal recall by 20 percent.

> People over age 70 and overweight showed less brain tissue in the frontal lobes, especially in the areas crucial to memory and planning, according to researchers at the University of Pittsburgh.

Pick perfect foods. Certain foods are not only good for you, they'll make it easier for you to lose pounds. Generally, choose fiber-rich grains, fruits, and vegetables. They help control your weight by filling you up faster and making you feel full longer. And eat foods that have fewer calories per serving. These are called low-energy-dense foods, which means you can eat more and feel full, while taking in fewer calories. Examples are most fruits and vegetables, low-fat meat and dairy, cooked grains, beans, and some cereals.

Here's a sampling of other power foods — those that have a unique element or combination of nutrients that will help you drop inches.

- Nuts. Rich in protein, fiber, and unsaturated fats, they are most helpful when you let them replace unhealthy snacks or desserts rich in trans fats and refined carbohydrates. Women who ate nuts two or more times a week gained less weight than women who didn't eat them.

- Grapefruit. Eat half a grapefruit before each meal and you could shed pounds without doing anything else. Experts believe there's a chemical link between grapefruit and insulin levels. The smaller the insulin spike after a meal, the more efficiently you use food for energy and the less fat is stored in your body. There's something in grapefruit that helps control insulin. It may be a compound called naringin, which slows enzymes in the small intestine responsible for metabolizing some fats and carbohydrates.

> There's a simple thing you can do every day to help you lose weight — or keep from gaining it in the first place — and it takes less than a minute. What is this miracle activity? Stepping on your bathroom scale. People in a two-year study who weighed themselves every day lost twice as much weight as those who weighed themselves weekly.

- Dairy foods. Dairy protein, or casein, works on weight management in several ways. All proteins satisfy your hunger, but casein is a slow protein, which means it sits in your digestive system a little bit longer. This can also control your insulin response — a good thing for weight control. Choose low-fat dairy products so you avoid extra calories.

- Eggs. Pick an egg breakfast over a carbohydrate-rich one, like bagels, and you should feel fewer hunger pangs throughout the day. In a study out of Saint Louis University, the egg eaters lost more weight and more inches around their waist than those on a bagel breakfast. Experts believe the protein is responsible for quelling your appetite.

Get a handle on belly fat

Abdominal fat is the most dangerous kind, but it is often the easiest to lose. See if your tummy roll puts you in the danger zone. Wrap a tape measure around your waist, level with your hip bones. Exhale and make it snug but not tight. If you're a woman and measure more than 35 inches, talk to your doctor about what you can do to lose those inches. Men are at risk if they're over 40 inches.

Omega-3 fatty acids

fatty fish • seeds • nuts • canola oil • flaxseed oil

Omega-3 fatty acids are a type of healthy, polyunsaturated fatty acid (PUFA) your body needs in order to function properly. You can't make them, so you must get them through your diet. The main types of omega-3s are docosahexaenoic acid (DHA), eicosapentaenoic acid (EPA), and alpha-linolenic acid (ALA). DHA and EPA are found in certain kinds of seafood, mostly cold-water, fatty fish, and ALA comes from plants.

Discover the value of omega-3s. These fats are important because they play vital roles in fighting many health problems.

- Omega-3 fatty acids curb the amount of inflammatory chemicals you produce. In addition, your body takes an ingredient in fish oil and turns it into Resolvin D2, a substance that reduces inflammation.

- Healthy cells are basic to overall good health, and omega-3 fats help by keeping cell membranes durable yet flexible — able to allow nutrients in, waste materials out, and ensure that cells can communicate with each other.

- You need omega-3 fats to control how much and what kind of powerful hormone-like substances called prostaglandins your body produces. Different prostaglandins impact different body functions, like blood pressure, blood clotting, and inflammation.

Balance your fatty acids. Unless you get smart about the other types of PUFAs, you could be sabotaging your quest for better health. Get to know omega-6 fatty acids.

These fats, found in meats, milk, eggs, some vegetable oils, and fried or processed foods, are not necessarily bad for you, but because they can encourage inflammation, you must eat them in moderation. Unfortunately, most people get way more omega-6 fats than omega-3s. Balancing these two nutrients is more important than you might think.

A better ratio of fatty acids may keep your immune system healthy, ward off diseases, and reduce already-active inflammation. Achieve this by cutting down on deep-fried foods; replacing corn, safflower, soybean, and cottonseed oils with olive or canola oils; and eating fewer processed and fast foods.

Don't rely on shellfish, like lobster, clams, crab, and shrimp, for your healthy dose of omega-3 fatty acids. Although they give you a small amount of this good-for-you fat, they are also high in cholesterol.

Count your grams. So just how much omega-3 fatty acids do you need? Some experts recommend most people get about 7 to 11 grams each week. You'll read later about how much you should get if you suffer from certain health conditions.

Generally, people think they're getting more of certain nutrients than they really are. That's why you can now test for omega-3 levels in your blood. Called the omega-3 index, it gives the proportion of omega-3 fatty acids as a percentage of total fatty acids in your red blood cells.

The home test is easy, but it's still fairly new, fairly expensive, and test results are not standardized among laboratories. Your doctor's office or an independent lab can also order the test, but insurance probably won't cover it. That said, it could be a lifesaving moment if you're at risk of heart disease. Check out a couple of home tests at *www.genesmart.com*, *www.nutrasource.ca/NDI/DiagConsumer.aspx*, and *www.omegaquant.com*.

Read on to discover how fish and other omega-3-rich foods can lower your risk of dementia and stroke, as well as give you protection from age-related memory loss.

	Total Omega-3 fatty acids (mg)	EPA (mg)	DHA (mg)	ALA (mg)
Fish sources				
1 tablespoon cod liver oil	2,664	931	1,481	
3 oz. Atlantic farmed salmon	1,921	587	1,238	
4 oz. canned pink salmon	1,356	404	776	
3 oz. white tuna canned in water	808	198	535	
Plant sources				
1 tablespoon flaxseed oil	7,196			7,196
1 oz. walnuts	2,565			2,565
1 tablespoon ground flaxseeds	1,597			1,597
1 tablespoon canola oil	1,279			1,279

4 ways omega-3 fatty acids keep you sharp

Keep your brain vital as you age. The more foods rich in omega-3 fatty acids you eat throughout your life, the smarter you could be in your golden years. This healthy fat protects you from dementia and mental decline in two ways.

- High blood levels of C-reactive protein (CRP), a natural marker of inflammation, indicate a greater risk of Alzheimer's disease (AD). Because CRP is actually poisonous to nerves and nerve tissue, it could be directly responsible for cell death in your hippocampus, the part of your brain responsible for forming new memories and storing old ones. As a source of eicosapentaenoic acid (EPA) and docosahexaenoic acid (DHA), omega-3 fatty acids are a perfect weapon to fight this inflammation.

- Too much zinc can kill cells responsible for sending and receiving signals in your brain, a key feature of AD. But DHA has the ability to control the amount of this mineral and keep it from triggering a dangerous imbalance.

The evidence is compelling. Tracking close to 15,000 people in seven countries, researchers found the more fatty fish they ate, the less likely they were to develop dementia. Not surprisingly, red meat had the opposite effect. So don't just add fish to your menu, make sure it replaces less-healthy choices, like red meat. And this is one case

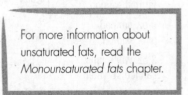

For more information about unsaturated fats, read the *Monounsaturated fats* chapter.

where a little fish goes a long way. Men who ate just one 5-ounce serving a week showed four times less mental decline over five years than men who didn't eat fish at all.

Hold on to your heart health. Anything that is bad for your heart and circulation is also bad for your brain. Stiff, clogged arteries mean less nutrient- and oxygen-rich blood circulates throughout your body. Clots within these arteries can mean a heart attack or stroke that kills brain cells. And high blood pressure can also trigger a stroke or reduce blood flow to your brain. Luckily, you can protect your heart from all these hazards with a single nutrient.

- Heart disease. Eat fish even if you don't have heart disease. In fact, the American Heart Association says eat it at least twice a week. It can reduce inflammation in your body and lower the levels of CRP in your blood, a risk factor for heart disease. Experts believe the components of omega-3 fatty acids work on the cellular level to improve blood pressure, your heart's electrical activity, and its muscle tone. If you have coronary heart disease, get about 1 gram (1,000 milligrams) of EPA and DHA daily, preferably from fish, although supplements are OK as long as you talk to your doctor first.

  > High amounts of omega-3 fatty acids through supplements could cause dangerous bleeding in some people. Talk to your doctor if you take more than 3 grams a day.

- Heart attack. As your blood level of omega-3 fatty acids goes up, your risk of sudden death from a heart attack goes down. A review of studies following nearly 40,000 people found those with heart disease should get a daily dose of about 1 gram of DHA and EPA to fend off a heart attack.

- Stroke. In a 14-year study of almost 80,000 women, those who enjoyed one fish entree at least twice a week cut their risk of stroke in half, compared to women who ate less fish.

- High cholesterol. Omega-3 fatty acids fight stiff, clogged arteries by lowering bad cholesterol and boosting the good. Interestingly enough, different sources impact cholesterol levels in different ways. ALA-rich walnuts, for instance, lower total and LDL cholesterol, while fatty fish lowers triglycerides and raises HDL cholesterol. Experts at the American Heart Association say if you need to lower your triglycerides, talk to your doctor about taking a supplement of 2 to 4 grams of EPA plus DHA every day.

Fight the funk of depression. Want to be happier? It could be as simple as eating foods rich in omega-3 fatty acids. Experts have known for years that cultures with high-fish diets suffer less from major depression, and people with major depression generally have low levels of omega-3 fatty acids. But until recently, there weren't good population studies to prove it. Then, in 2010, university researchers published results from the largest study ever on omega-3s for depression, finding the fatty acid improved symptoms as well as prescription antidepressants. There are a few ways this could work.

> Salmon is the perfect package for a brighter mood, better sleep, and stronger memory. Not only is it chock-full of omega-3 fatty acids, which are like nature's antidepressant, but it also contains magnesium and vitamin B12.

- Suffering from chronic, low-grade inflammation is a risk factor for depression. As an anti-inflammatory, omega-3 fatty acids, especially from fish oils, can lessen this risk.

- Polyunsaturated fats, like omega-3s, are known to control signals between neurons and influence how cells respond to specific signals. These signals often pass on information related to emotions.

- Not enough fatty acid in your brain could mean an imbalance of brain chemicals that influence mood.

This groundbreaking study used 1,050 milligrams (mg) of EPA and 150 mg of DHA every day. To get these omega-3 components through diet, eat fatty fish like bluefin tuna, Atlantic wild salmon, mackerel, wild rainbow trout, and herring.

Slim you down. It's no fairy tale. There are delicious foods that can work behind-the-scenes magic to help you lose weight.

- Fat equals stored energy. Too much fat equals more pounds because you're storing too much energy. That's why working off energy through exercise helps you lose weight. Omega-3 fatty acids do the same thing from the inside out, boosting the production of heat by burning energy, a process called thermogenesis.

- It's easier to stop eating if you're not hungry. By changing the levels of hunger hormones, like ghrelin and leptin, omega-3s help you feel full after a meal.

An Australian study reports that overweight and obese people had lower omega-3 blood levels than people of a healthy weight. And the flip side was true — people with higher omega-3 levels generally had healthier weights, and smaller waist and hip sizes, suggesting this fatty acid can be especially important in shrinking dangerous belly fat.

Top tips to avoid fish dangers

Large, predatory fish may contain contaminants like mercury and PCBs (polychlorinated biphenyls). But don't let this scare you away from getting a healthy dose of omega-3 fatty acids. Unless you're pregnant or very young, the benefits of eating fish far outweigh the potential risks. Just learn to make smart choices.

- Eat a variety of fish to reduce your risk of exposure to contaminants.

- Avoid tilefish, shark, swordfish, and king mackerel. These have the highest levels of mercury.

- Remove the skin and surface fat from risky fish before cooking.

- Many health professionals say it's safe to eat 14 ounces a week of fish with mercury levels that average 0.5 parts per million. That includes fresh or frozen tuna, red snapper, and orange roughy.

Eat like the Greeks for super health

A delicious combination of healthy foods really shouldn't be called a diet — yet the Mediterranean diet, based on foods native to Greece and southern Italy, is the way to go if you want to slay a slew of health problems. Emphasizing whole grains, fresh fruits and vegetables, olive oil, nuts, legumes, and fish rich in omega-3 fatty acids, the Mediterranean diet has proven to be amazingly effective in keeping you sharp into your golden years.

By working against inflammation, high cholesterol, increased blood pressure, and oxidative damage from free radicals, this eating plan could:

- slash the danger of heart attack by 50 percent.

- lower your risk of developing Alzheimer's disease (AD) by 40 percent.

- decrease the odds that mild mental impairment will progress to AD.

- help people with diabetes achieve better glycemic control.

- help you lose weight more than traditional low-fat diets.

For more information about the Mediterranean diet, see the *Age-related macular degeneration* chapter.

Parkinson's disease

tremors • stooped posture • slow movement
• poor balance • shuffling walk
• depression • anxiety • dementia

When you think of Parkinson's disease, you probably think of the actor Michael J. Fox, whose public battle with the disease has focused attention on it. But you should also think of your brain — and how to protect it.

Main symptoms of Parkinson's disease include tremors, stooped posture, slow movement, poor balance, and a shuffling walk. But Parkinson's doesn't just affect your movements. It can also affect your thinking, memory, language, and problem-solving skills. You may even experience depression, anxiety, dementia, or paranoia.

Gout can be a real pain, but a compound linked to gout may reduce your risk of Parkinson's disease. Uric acid may protect your brain's neurons from oxidative stress with its antioxidant properties. Foods that boost uric acid include anchovies, herring, mackerel, mussels, organ meats, and gravy. Just don't go overboard — or you could end up with gout.

That's because of what's happening in your brain. While no one knows for sure what causes Parkinson's, the main feature of the disease is a loss of dopamine, a key neurotransmitter that affects movement, coordination, and information processing. Changes in the brain may also impair the release of norepinephrine, another important brain chemical.

Protein deposits called Lewy bodies show up in the brains of people with Parkinson's disease. Lewy bodies may kill nerve cells or simply be the byproduct of degeneration.

You can't do much about many Parkinson's risk factors — including age, race, gender, and genetic factors — but you can try to limit others. For instance, middle-age weight gain, diabetes, and exposure to pesticides and herbicides have been linked to increased risk of Parkinson's.

The drug levodopa, which is converted to dopamine in your brain, is the standard treatment for Parkinson's disease. Treatment may also include other medications and procedures, including deep brain stimulation. This involves implanting electrodes in your brain and a battery pack in your chest. The steady electrical current helps control symptoms of Parkinson's. But you can also take some less-drastic steps to prevent and manage the disease.

5 tactics to fight Parkinson's disease

Choose vitamins that help. Get enough of these important vitamins, and you could get a jump on preventing Parkinson's disease.

- Vitamin E. A diet rich in this antioxidant vitamin could protect you from Parkinson's, according to a Canadian study. Opt for vitamin E from food sources, such as green leafy vegetables, seeds, nuts, and olive oil, rather than supplements.

- Vitamin D. Emory University researchers discovered that people with Parkinson's disease were more likely to have insufficient levels of vitamin D than healthy people or those with Alzheimer's disease. Because of mobility problems, people with Parkinson's might get less sun exposure, which could explain the deficiency. But low vitamin D levels may also contribute to Parkinson's and boosting your intake may help.

- Vitamin B6. A Dutch study found that getting more vitamin B6 into your diet may decrease your risk of Parkinson's. This could be because it plays a key role in the production of dopamine. You can find vitamin B6 in dark leafy greens, seafood, legumes, whole grains, and fruits and vegetables.

Reach for coffee or tea. Whether you prefer coffee or tea, you can protect your brain from Parkinson's. If you really like coffee, you'll really like this news. According to a Finnish study, drinking 10 cups of coffee a day can slash your risk by a whopping 84 percent. Other research suggests that even one cup a day can cut your risk in half. The caffeine in coffee may help by stimulating dopamine.

Just as with coffee, more tea means more protection. A Chinese study found that people who drank at least 23 cups of black tea a month had a 71 percent lower risk of developing Parkinson's disease than those who drank less. While caffeine was associated with a lower risk of Parkinson's, black tea's other ingredients, including its complex antioxidants, seem to provide the protection. In animal tests, the polyphenols found in green tea also show promise for fighting Parkinson's.

It takes two to tango, and this dance may be just what it takes to help people with Parkinson's disease. A recent Washington University study found that tango lessons improved mobility and balance in people with Parkinson's. In fact, any kind of dancing provides benefits. Just play your favorite music and move to the beat.

Limit potential links. Not all food and beverages have a protective effect. You may want to enjoy some foods in moderation. A recent study found that men who consumed a lot of dairy products — especially milk — were much more likely to develop Parkinson's disease. Researchers can't explain why or why the link only applies to men.

High intakes of iron and manganese have also been linked to Parkinson's. One study found that people whose diets contained a lot of iron from plant sources, like fortified cereals and grains, were 30 percent more likely to develop the disease. Iron could contribute to Parkinson's by causing oxidative damage in the brain.

Try tai chi. This low-impact, slow-motion exercise could be just what the doctor ordered. One small study found that tai chi improved balance, walking ability, and overall well-being in people with mild to moderately severe Parkinson's disease. Other people benefit from Pilates, which increases core strength, flexibility, and balance. But any regular exercise should help.

Relieve pain and reduce risk. Taking aspirin and other nonsteroidal anti-inflammatory drugs, like ibuprofen, may lessen your risk. A recent study determined that people who took these pain relievers at least twice a week for a month or more were less likely to develop Parkinson's. Interestingly, aspirin helped women, but not men. Talk with your doctor before taking aspirin or another NSAID regularly.

Precautions to take when taking drugs

Drugs can help control symptoms of Parkinson's disease, but they also come with their own risks. Be aware of these potential dangers.

Levodopa. Dietary protein can interfere with levodopa, the most common drug for Parkinson's. You can improve the medication's effectiveness by taking it 45 minutes before meals with a cracker. You may also want to limit your protein intake during the day.

Anticholinergics. These drugs, which are sometimes used to treat Parkinson's, may harm your memory. They work by blocking the binding of the brain chemical acetylcholine to its receptor in nerve cells. But you need acetylcholine for a good memory. Regular use of anticholinergics may hamper your ability to perform daily tasks, such as shopping or managing your money. If you are taking one of these drugs, ask your doctor if you need to continue.

Pergolide and cabergoline. Known as dopamine agonists, they mimic the effect of dopamine in your brain. They are sometimes prescribed for Parkinson's and may damage your heart valves. Ask your doctor about switching medications and getting an echocardiogram to check for damage.

Recall strategies

focus • get organized • use your senses • say it out loud • write it down • make a mnemonic • visualize • doodle • relax • enjoy nature

"Memory is a net; one finds it full of fish when he takes it from the brook; but a dozen miles of water have run through it without sticking." Oliver Wendell Holmes, Sr., 19th century American poet and medical doctor, may have been more right than he knew.

The hippocampus, a small, S-shaped part of the brain, plays a major role in memory formation. It reviews all the information flowing in from your five senses and decides which bits to keep and which to throw away. The hippocampus itself doesn't store any memories. These get tucked away in different areas of your brain.

Scientists used to think you had two main types of memory — long-term and short-term. Now they know you have at least four.

Episodic. What did you eat for dinner last night, and what did you talk about? Episodic memory helps you recall personal experiences like this. When this area fails, you may struggle to learn new information or remember recent events.

Semantic. This stores general facts and knowledge, like the number of days in a week, the difference between a fork and a comb, and the name of the first president of the United States. People who have trouble naming or describing a common object may have a problem with their semantic memory.

Procedural. This type of memory played a big part in your childhood. It enabled you to learn things that eventually became automatic, like how to tie your shoelaces or ride a bicycle. If you forget how to do tasks you had once mastered or have serious problems learning new skills, procedural memory could be to blame.

Working. You can think of this as your "short-term memory." It controls your ability to concentrate, pay attention, and temporarily store information, like directions or a phone number. People who struggle to concentrate or learn a task with multiple steps may have trouble with their working memory.

Don't panic over an occasional lapse in one of these areas. Everyone forgets things, especially when they are tired, sick, distracted, or under stress. Even when your brain is firing on all cylinders, you will store and recall some memories more easily than others. That said, science does link certain health problems, such as the ones that follow, with specific types of memory loss.

Sharpen your brain with chewing gum. Smacking a stick of sugar-free gum may improve your memory and help you stay focused. Eighth-graders who chewed gum during math class, while doing homework, and during tests did better in math class and on standardized math tests than kids who didn't get gum. Experts say gum chewing may ease stress and anxiety and improve concentration.

Condition	Type of memory affected			
	Episodic	Semantic	Procedural	Working
Normal aging				✔
Alzheimer's disease	✔	✔		✔
Mild cognitive impairment	✔			
Lewy body dementia	✔			✔
Vascular dementia	✔			✔
Medication side effects	✔			✔
Vitamin B12 deficiency	✔			✔
Hypoglycemia	✔			
Anxiety	✔			
Depression			✔	
Obsessive-compulsive disorder			✔	✔
Cardiopulmonary bypass	✔			✔
Multiple sclerosis	✔			✔
Parkinson's disease			✔	✔
Traumatic brain injury	✔	✔		✔

11 recall strategies that keep you sharp

Reject negative beliefs about aging. Believing that your memory will get worse with age may actually make it happen. Negative stereotypes like this about aging can worsen your ability to remember things.

Researchers tested the memories of seniors from 60 to 82 years old and suggested to some of them that older people have worse memories than younger people. Those who heard this, especially the younger seniors, tended to do worse on memory tests than the others. So the next time someone tells you memory fades with age, tell them "you're only as old, or as young, as you think."

Pay attention. Stop trying to do two things at once if you hope to remember them. Your brain needs to focus on information for about eight seconds in order to process and store it in the right memory center. Dividing your attention among several tasks at one time makes this harder. Boost your recall by focusing on the item or information, and block out distractions as best you can.

Get organized. It's easy to forget things when you're surrounded by clutter. Start by organizing the place where you keep your notes, calendar, to-do lists, and phone numbers. You will feel less flustered when you can lay your hands on important information quickly.

Move your eyes from side to side after learning something new, and you may be more likely to remember it. People were asked to study lists of words and then shift their gaze either side to side or up and down for 30 seconds, or do nothing. Those who looked side to side remembered more words off the list and were less likely to imagine seeing words that weren't there.

Next, get your mind in order. Don't try to remember lots of tidbits of information, like grocery and to-do lists. Write these down instead and post them on your refrigerator or in another prominent place. Or buy an inexpensive appointment book to carry with you. Look for one with a calendar, note pad, and directory to write down phone numbers.

Create a habit. Make a task mindless, and you'll be less likely to forget it. For instance, set a basket on the counter as a catchall for keys and wallets, and drop them there as soon as you walk in the door. Designate a place to put things you often lose, like eyeglasses or TV remotes, and then stow them there every time. You will never again wonder where they are.

Engage your senses. Put your senses of taste, touch, smell, sight, and hearing to work. Experts say the more senses you use in making a memory, the more of your brain is involved in storing it. The next time you're in a situation you want to capture, stop and notice the sounds, sights, and smells around you.

Repeat it. You may look as though you're talking to yourself, but repeating things out loud will help you remember them. As soon as you meet someone new, use their name in conversation to help it stick in your memory. The same trick works when you read or think of something you need to remember. "I am locking the door" can remind you that you locked up the house before heading to bed. Writing down information with your own hand serves a similar purpose.

Make a mnemonic. You probably remember what "ROY G BIV" stands for, even after all these years (red, orange, yellow, green, blue, indigo, violet). Mnemonics, or memory tricks, like this one can help you remember everything from the grocery list to your grandkids' names.

- Acronyms use the first letter of each word in a phrase to form a new word, like ROY G BIV or NOAA (National Oceanic and Atmospheric Administration). Write out the first letter of each item on your grocery list and try arranging them into a word you can remember.

- Acrostics also use the first letter of each word, but turn them into a nonsense sentence. For instance, "Every Good Boy Does Fine" represents the notes E, G, B, D, and F on the treble clef in music.

- Rhymes can make even hard-to-remember facts catchy. Who could forget the classic, "30 days has September, April, June, and November?" Coming up with your own rhymes can be a challenge. Make a game out of it with your spouse to see who can think up the funniest phrases.

- Alliteration — when words begin with the same letter or sound — works great for remembering names and places, like the fact that you're meeting "Chatty Cathy" at the "delicious deli" this afternoon.

Use your imagination. Pairing a visual image with someone's name will help it stick for next time. When you meet someone for the first time, create an image in your mind that seems to match their name. Rosalyn might be a rose, while Bill is a baseball cap. Be sure to choose a pleasant image. The mind tends to block out negative ones.

Relax. Stress and anxiety don't do your brain any favors. Ask any college student who has studied for hours only to draw a blank during a big test. Slow down and relax when learning something you need to remember. Techniques such as deep breathing and muscle relaxation exercises can help boost your recall naturally.

Draw doodles. It's simple and mindless, but it may help you remember. Researchers tested people's memories by asking them to listen to a boring phone conversation with lots of names and places. Half were told to doodle while listening. During tests, doodlers recalled nearly 30 percent more names and places. Experts think this mindless activity helps keep you awake and alert during boring tasks and cuts down on daydreaming, which takes your attention away from matters at hand.

Get out in nature. Being in nature, even looking at nature photos, can improve your memory and attention. Nature captures your attention but doesn't require much thought, giving tired brains a rest. City surroundings, however, demand high levels of attention with car horns, billboards, and traffic. The next time you need a mental break or a memory boost, take a stroll outdoors among the trees and flowers, or sit down with a gardening or bird-watching magazine.

7 habits of people with the sharpest memories

Ever forget someone's name a moment after you meet them? How embarrassing. You can be the life of the party with these simple strategies. All are easy and pleasant to do.

Try rhythm and rhyme. Use rhyme or alliteration to make a name stick in your head. A perky Betsy could be "Bouncy Betsy" and a gloomy Daniel "Dour Dan."

Concentrate. Focus your attention as you are introduced, to help your brain process and store the memory.

Use it or lose it. Repeat the person's name back to them soon after you hear it, with a comment like, "Hi Dan. It's so nice to meet you."

Spell it out. Ask the person to clarify the spelling of their name. For instance, "Is that Jerry with a J or a G?" Then see the letters in your head.

Put it in writing. Write down the name if you are able. The act of putting it on paper helps imprint it on your brain.

Make mental connections. Relate the name to something or someone else you know, like an overweight Henry to King Henry VIII.

Get creative. Match hard-to-remember names with images. Imagine "John Zuderman" wearing a red cape just like Super Man to remind you his last name sounds similar.

Resistance training

sharpens your mind • prevents falls
• fends off frailty • fights fat • controls blood sugar
• battles high blood pressure

The tiny, 98-year-old woman on the local news still lives independently. She's as sharp as a tack and does her own shopping, housework, and yard work. Her secret weapon — resistance training. It can be a powerful weapon for you, too.

Resistance training, sometimes called strength training or weight lifting, means you improve your muscle strength by gradually improving your muscles' ability to push back against extra weight or an outside force. You can do this three ways — lifting free weights, like barbells; using resistance bands or weight machines; or using your own body weight as you do in push-ups.

Resistance training is important because your muscle cells start to waste away if you don't use your muscles often enough. But when you start strength training, you create harmless tears in your muscles.

These tears are larger versions of the wear and tear from daily living, but they are so tiny you can't see them without a microscope. The tears alert your body's repair systems. If your muscles get enough rest and nutrition, the body repairs these tears by making the muscle slightly larger and a whole lot stronger. This makes the muscle more resistant to stress and damage.

But you must do resistance training regularly or your muscles can begin to waste away again. What's more, as your muscles become stronger and more stress-resistant, you must add extra weight to your exercises to make sure you reap all the benefits of resistance training.

5 ways resistance training keeps you sharp

Prevents falls and frailty. You can stop the #1 cause of your body's deterioration. Sarcopenia is the gradual loss of muscle strength that naturally happens as you grow older. It can begin as early as age 40 and may lead to frailty, loss of independence, and a higher risk of falls. That risk of falls may be particularly dangerous because falls are a leading cause of brain injury. According to research, head injury raises your risk of mental decline, including Alzheimer's disease and other forms of dementia.

But studies also suggest resistance training can help stop age-related muscle loss. For example, one study found that people over age 65 who took up resistance training gained back some of the strength they had lost, but that's not all. They actually reversed age-related changes in their muscle cells, too. What's more, strength training slashes your risk of falls and helps you stay strong enough to perform the daily tasks of living, so you can keep living independently for years to come.

Helps control your blood sugar. Several studies suggest that resistance training can help insulin control your blood sugar. Muscle cells naturally take in and use plenty of blood sugar. But resistance training improves your muscles' ability to store glucose, so even less glucose gets left in your bloodstream.

That may be why one study found that less insulin was needed to control blood sugar in people who did resistance training. You need that kind of protection because your body tends to over-produce insulin as diabetes develops.

Research shows that men who do not produce the right amount of insulin at age 50 face a significantly greater risk of developing Alzheimer's disease and other types of dementia later on.

> For best results, each exercise should take around seven seconds. Spend three seconds lifting the weight into position, one second holding it in place, and three more seconds lowering the weight to the position where it started.

Battles obesity and belly fat. According to one study, people who were obese at middle age were three times more likely to develop Alzheimer's disease than people at a healthy weight. This may happen because fat cells produce dangerous inflammatory compounds that travel into your brain.

A German study found that people who cut calories and lost weight scored better on memory tests. Recent studies suggest resistance training can decrease your percentage of body fat, help you avoid gaining belly fat, and prevent weight gain after you've lost it. Adding more muscle may make weight loss even easier because muscle burns three times as many calories as fat.

Fends off dementia and memory loss. Lifting weights for one hour twice a week can help you focus in spite of distractions, make better decisions, and resolve conflicts, a recent study found. Researchers suspect that resistance training may reduce beta-amyloid in brain tissues. Beta-amyloid is a key ingredient in the brain plaques associated with Alzheimer's disease.

Defends against heart attacks and strokes. Obesity and high blood sugar may raise your risk of heart disease. When you take up resistance training to help control your weight and blood sugar, you are taking a powerful step to resist heart disease, too.

What's more, preliminary studies suggest resistance training may help lower "bad" LDL cholesterol and trim high blood pressure. This exercise can even help people with heart disease keep or regain the strength to do daily activities. Unfortunately, standard resistance training may not be safe for people with uncontrolled high blood pressure or other heart or artery problems, so talk with your doctor before you try it. But don't give up hope. Experts suggest a doctor-guided,

Check with your doctor before you begin resistance training — especially if you smoke, have had recent surgery, are sedentary, or have a serious health condition, such as osteoporosis, asthma, cancer, chronic back or joint problems, high blood pressure, or heart disease. You may need a resistance training program customized for you.

modified version of resistance training may have significant benefits for many people with heart disease.

Smart tips for first-timers

You can start resistance training even if you are sedentary or over age 70. Just remember to start slowly and follow these rules.

- Do resistance exercises for all your major muscle groups — chest, back, legs, arms, shoulders, and abdominals — on two days of the week for 30 minutes, but never two days in a row.

- Avoid weights that are too heavy. If your physical condition is poor when you first start, practice the exercises with no weights or with 1- or 2-pound weights. If you cannot push or lift a weight eight times, switch to a lighter weight.

- Learn the lingo. Each time you do strength-training exercises, such as arm curls, it is called a repetition or rep. Fifteen arm curls equals 15 reps. A group of reps makes a set. For example, 15 reps of arm curls is one set. If you rest and then do 15 more arm curls, that is your second set. When you begin resistance training, set a goal to complete one set or 10 to 15 reps of each exercise. You may not reach your goal right away, but do as many as you can.

- Never hold your breath during a resistance exercise. Instead, breathe out as you lift and breathe in as you relax.

- Avoid jerking the weights. Move them steadily and slowly.

- Soup cans, vegetable cans, bagged rice, or bottled water can serve as hand weights.

- Warm up with five to 10 minutes of light aerobic exercise, such as walking, before every training session. Finish each workout with five minutes of cool-down stretches.

Beware of these warning signs

Most people have sore muscles during the first weeks of resistance training, but stop exercising and check with your doctor if you have these symptoms.

- sharp or severe pains in your bones, joints, feet, ankles, or legs

- fever from a cold, flu, or infection

- fatigue that is much worse than usual

- a swollen or painful muscle or joint

- any new or unexplained symptom

If you experience chest, neck, shoulder or arm pain or pressure; breathing trouble; lightheadedness; dizziness; nausea; or break out in a cold sweat, call your doctor immediately.

Resveratrol

grapes • red wine • grape juice • raisins • cocoa
• dark chocolate • peanuts • peanut butter • blueberries
• cranberries • pomegranates

Next time you toast someone's health with a glass of red wine, consider toasting the grape itself. That's because grapes contain resveratrol. This amazing compound, found in the skins, provides several health benefits.

Plants produce resveratrol to protect themselves from stress, injury, fungal infection, and the sun's ultraviolet rays. But it may also protect you from several harmful conditions.

Found mostly in grapes, red wine, grape juice, peanuts, and some berries, resveratrol has been studied for its beneficial effects on heart disease, cancer, and longevity. It has antioxidant, anti-inflammatory, and anti-clotting powers, and it works in a variety of ways. Several preliminary studies paint resveratrol as a promising treatment.

1 cup boiled peanuts	0.92 mg*
1 cup red grapes	0.745 mg
5-oz. glass grape juice	0.7 mg
5-oz. glass red wine	0.685 mg
2 tablespoons peanut butter	0.01 mg

* milligrams

So how much of this great substance do you need? Currently, there is no official recommended dietary allowance (RDA) or dietary reference intake (DRI) for resveratrol. But a recent report determined the "prudent intake" (PI) to be 0.49 milligrams a day, excluding wine. That same report found that 89 percent of adults fall short of this goal. It should be noted that the report was funded by Nutrilite, a leading manufacturer of dietary supplements.

One advantage supplements have over food is they give you a set dose of resveratrol. Whether you drink grape juice or eat grapes, it's difficult to know exactly how much resveratrol you're getting. Amounts vary widely, depending on the type of grape, region, soil, method of storage, and other factors.

But that doesn't mean you shouldn't try to boost your dietary intake of this important compound, especially since whole foods provide key nutrients and phytonutrients besides resveratrol. However you get your resveratrol, you — and your brain — will be getting quite a boost. Cheers!

4 ways resveratrol keeps you sharp

Fends off dementia. To keep your mind from slipping, do some sipping. Epidemiological studies suggest moderate red wine consumption — one glass a day for women and up to two a day for men — helps lower the incidence of Alzheimer's disease and other forms of dementia. In fact, drinking wine may be even more protective than taking nonsteroidal anti-inflammatory drugs (NSAIDs).

The resveratrol in red wine likely accounts for these positive results. Recent studies have explored the effects of resveratrol on the brain — and revealed several ways it may help.

One way is by thwarting beta-amyloid, the protein that forms plaques in the brains of people with Alzheimer's disease. In lab studies, resveratrol lowers the levels of beta-amyloid in cell cultures. While resveratrol does not limit production of beta-amyloid, it does spark its breakdown.

In a Cornell study of mice, resveratrol diminished beta-amyloid plaque formation in certain regions of the brain. Researchers aren't sure how it works, but suspect it may have something to do with an accompanying increase in cysteine and decrease in glutathione, chemicals found in the brain.

Researchers at Rensselaer Polytechnic Institute found that resveratrol can neutralize the toxic effects of proteins linked to Alzheimer's disease. Resveratrol seems to target specific proteins and rearrange them so they become nontoxic to human cells.

Resveratrol can give even healthy brains a boost. British researchers recently discovered that resveratrol increases blood flow to the brain when people perform mental tasks.

Although red wine and resveratrol have not been proven to prevent dementia, they show tremendous promise.

Pumps up your heart. What's good for your heart is often good for your brain. So take heart from research that suggests resveratrol can help keep your ticker ticking.

Evidence for red wine first surfaced when researchers took note of the "French Paradox." French people often eat high-fat foods, smoke, and drink wine, yet they have low rates of heart disease. The key, many experts say, is red wine.

Recent studies shed more light on how resveratrol, a key component of red wine, may help your heart. Chronic inflammation contributes to several conditions, including heart disease and brain disorders, and resveratrol fights inflammation. It also helps prevent platelets from clumping and clotting.

One study found that resveratrol sparks new blood vessel growth in rats after a heart attack. This helps maintain blood flow to the heart when an artery is blocked. Another laboratory study determined that resveratrol tames cells that contribute to cardiac fibrosis, or stiffening of the heart muscle, and hamper your heart's ability to contract.

Look out and listen up! In addition to your brain, resveratrol may also protect your eyes and ears. Resveratrol can stop out-of-control blood vessel growth in your eyes. This abnormal blood vessel growth contributes to diabetic retinopathy and age-related macular degeneration, conditions that can cause blindness. Resveratrol also shields your ears from noise-induced hearing loss.

Fights fat. A big belly means a big risk for heart disease, diabetes, and even dementia. Gobbling some grapes may help keep you in shape. Research indicates that resveratrol helps combat obesity.

A German lab study found that resveratrol reduces the number of fat cells by preventing pre-fat cells from increasing and converting into mature fat cells. It also blocks the production of certain chemicals called cytokines linked to the development of obesity-related disorders, such as diabetes and clogged arteries.

Researchers at the University of Georgia reached similar results. Resveratrol not only prevented pre-fat cells from growing, it also triggered apoptosis, or cell death, in mature fat cells.

University of New Mexico researchers found that resveratrol reduces inflammation in fat tissue. That's important because chronic, low-level inflammation in fat tissue contributes to heart disorders and insulin resistance, a pre-cursor to diabetes.

Resveratrol also works in animal studies. In a French study of lemurs, resveratrol decreased energy intake by 13 percent and boosted the resting metabolic rate by 29 percent. In other words, lemurs ate less and burned calories faster — a great recipe for weight loss. Perhaps most interesting, resveratrol mimics caloric restriction in mice. This means it tricks your body into thinking it's getting fewer calories. Previous studies showed that caloric restriction extends the life span of mice.

> Nibble on some chocolate, and you'll get a sweet surprise — a healthy dose of resveratrol. Researchers in Hershey, Pa., found that cocoa powder trails only red wine and grape juice among foods with the highest resveratrol content. You'll get the most resveratrol from cocoa powder, followed by unsweetened baking chocolate, semi-sweet chocolate chips, dark chocolate, milk chocolate, and chocolate syrup.

Benefits blood sugar. Here's some sweet news for people with diabetes — resveratrol may help improve your blood sugar levels. Managing diabetes also helps lower the risk of heart disease and dementia.

In an Indian study, resveratrol lowered blood sugar and improved the levels of insulin and hemoglobin in diabetic rats. These results were similar to those achieved by glyclazide, a diabetes drug taken by mouth, making resveratrol a promising treatment for diabetes. Turkish researchers found that resveratrol improved glucose metabolism and relaxed the blood vessels in diabetic rats.

A recent study found that resveratrol lowers blood sugar levels by helping it move into certain tissues, including skeletal muscle.

Resveratrol can even help soothe some of the complications of diabetes. Another study found that resveratrol helps relieve the pain of diabetic neuropathy, or nerve damage caused by high blood sugar levels.

Smart supplement strategies

Shopping for resveratrol supplements can be a challenge. Whether you browse store shelves or search online, you'll find plenty of options — and plenty of confusion.

How much should you take, for instance? In animal studies, researchers often use very large amounts — the equivalent of about 2 grams for people. But that is likely too high. One expert recommends about 5 milligrams (mg) per kilogram of body weight, or about 350 mg a day for an average adult.

When reading labels, be aware that some products list the amount of resveratrol in micrograms (mcg) rather than mg. It may look like a whopping dose of resveratrol, but it takes 1,000 mcg to equal 1 mg.

Also pay attention to the type of resveratrol in the supplement. It comes in two main forms, trans-resveratrol and cis-resveratrol. Opt for trans-resveratrol, the more stable and effective form. Choose capsules over tablets. Because resveratrol is prone to oxidation, the tablets may lose effectiveness over time.

If you're taking blood-thinning drugs, you may want to avoid resveratrol because of its anti-platelet activity.

Because of a lack of human trials, it's not even clear if

> Sip your red wine slowly. Not only does that allow you to savor it, but it also helps you absorb more resveratrol. Resveratrol becomes largely inactivated by your gut or liver, but it can reach your bloodstream through the mucous membranes in your mouth.

resveratrol supplements do any good. While they seem safe, the long-term effects remain a mystery. Always talk to your doctor before taking any supplements.

Perks and perils of drinking alcohol

When it comes to alcohol, think small. This beverage can protect your brain cells — or it can kill them. The key is the amount.

In a study of more than 3,000 people age 75 and older, those who had one or two drinks a day had a 40 percent lower risk of developing dementia. However, for those who already had mild mental impairment at the start of the study, moderate drinking did not help. And heavy drinking — more than two drinks a day — boosted the risk of progressing into dementia.

An Australian review of 15 studies also found that moderate drinking reduces the risk of Alzheimer's disease and other forms of dementia for people over age 60.

If you don't drink, don't start just for the potential brain benefits. But if you do drink, limit your intake to one or two drinks a day.

Annual deaths	Alcohol prevented	Alcohol caused
100,000		
50,000		other cardiovascular disease
		liver disease
		cancer
25,000	heart disease	pancreatitis
	stroke	overdose
	diabetes	injury

Peanut-crusted chicken is a variation of a popular Asian dish — peanut pork. This recipe is high in protein, low in fat, and gives you a dose of resveratrol with its crunchy peanut coating.

Peanut-crusted chicken

4 boneless, skinless chicken breast fillets
1 cup salted peanuts
2 tbsp. canola oil
4 tbsp. honey

Using a blender or coffee grinder, reduce the peanuts to a coarse mixture. Do not over grind or you will end up with dry peanut butter.

Lightly salt and pepper the chicken breast fillets and brush on a coating of honey for binding and flavor. Place the chicken in the coarsely chopped peanuts and press the coating into the chicken with the back of a tablespoon.

Coat a deep frying pan with the canola oil and heat on high. Place the chicken in the skillet, reduce heat to medium, and cook until golden brown, 30 to 45 minutes.

This dish can also be baked, eliminating the canola oil. Bake the fillets at 350 degrees for 45 minutes or until crusty brown on top. Slice and serve piping hot as an entree, or serve it with your favorite dipping sauce as an appetizer.

Makes 4 servings

Sleep disorders

difficulty falling asleep • interrupted sleep • tingling legs
• disrupted breathing • snoring

Memories are made of protein. Not quite the lyrics of a romantic song, but stirring stuff in the world of neuroscience. In fact, the first Nobel Prize of the 21st century went to the discovery of a protein that hooks up with your DNA to switch on the memory-making process.

Scientists know the human brain doesn't work exactly like a computer, where information is automatically stored on a hard drive. Something has to actually trigger the storage process. And this protein-based theory explains how it happens on a molecular level. It's proven if you block the ability to make new proteins, your brain simply cannot turn a task, thought, idea, or process into a long-term memory. So what does this have to do with sleep?

When something happens during your day, you can hold onto it for a few hours without any special protein action in your brain. In order to turn it into a long-term memory, your body must go through what's called a circadian cycle, or a 24-hour period of sleep, wakefulness, and other biological activities. This cycle is important for the proteins to do their job. During sleep, memories are strengthened and integrated into the part of your brain responsible for forming new memories and storing long-term ones.

Recent research has revealed that even mild to moderate sleep loss can have devastating effects on thinking and memory. In one study, people who got only six hours of sleep a night were slower to react, couldn't think as clearly, and performed poorly on simple memory tasks.

If you're worried about basic brainpower, catching enough Z's is an essential tool. Sleep loss means sluggish reaction time, inability to make decisions, difficulty processing information, more negative emotions, and a lousy mood.

If you simply need to amp up your creative thinking, make sure you get some REM (rapid eye movement) sleep. This stage occurs about 90 minutes after you fall asleep. During this time, your heart rate and respiration speed up, your eyes move rapidly, and you dream intensely. A University of California, San Diego study showed REM sleep improved creative problem-solving skills by almost 40 percent.

Because sharp thinking is also related to overall health, consider how sleep impacts you in other ways.

High blood pressure. To keep a good supply of oxygen-rich blood flowing to your brain, you need wide-open, flexible arteries — much like a congestion-free highway system keeps traffic moving steadily. There's a definite but unexplained association between enough quality sleep and heart health.

People who don't get the necessary 40 winks are more likely to have high blood pressure, and if they go to bed after midnight, they're more likely to have stiffer arteries, an early stage of hardening of the arteries or atherosclerosis. But in a five-year study of middle-age adults, an extra hour of sleep each night reduced plaque buildup in their arteries by 33 percent.

> Learn a lesson from 56 students who participated in a recent sleep study. The students who studied, then slept, then were tested did better than those who hadn't slept. And even if it appears you've forgotten things you learned during the day, a good night's sleep can restore your memories.

Diabetes. This disease can attack your brain power with its short-term symptoms and its long-term complications. And now groundbreaking research may explain the link between this condition and poor sleep, which translates into a lack of blood sugar control. In fact, people who sleep less than six hours a night are almost five times more likely to develop abnormal fasting blood sugar levels. New studies explain that the hormone melatonin, which is closely tied to your body's sleep clock, may also directly control insulin production.

Obesity. Extra weight and its connection to heart disease and obesity is hazardous to your memory. People who don't get enough sleep are more likely to weigh more, carry more dangerous fat around their middle, and eat more fat-laden foods. There are several possible explanations for this. If you're sleep-deprived, an imbalance of the hormones leptin and ghrelin may make you feel hungrier. And since you're awake longer, you've got more opportunities to eat. On the other hand, you may feel tired and less likely to exercise, which also contributes to weight gain.

> It's more difficult for you to remember a new task if you don't sleep within 30 hours of learning it.

4 tactics to fight sleep disorders

Uncover the cause of insomnia. This is the first of several preventable and treatable conditions that can keep you from a good night's sleep. Insomnia, by definition, is difficulty falling asleep and staying asleep. It can be both a condition and a symptom. Talk with your doctor if you have trouble sleeping. She may want to rule out any number of things, like anxiety or depression, that could be causing your trouble.

In the meantime, there are several lifestyle changes you can make on your own to help you spend more time in dreamland.

- Get some exercise every day.

- Avoid caffeine and alcohol, which can disrupt your sleep.

- Adapt your sleep environment and bedtime rituals so you're relaxed. Learn more about this in the *Sleep strategies* chapter.

- Spend some time outdoors in the morning sunshine to set your body's clock.

- Practice relaxation techniques, like deep breathing, gentle stretching, and quiet time.

Manage sleep apnea. If you stop breathing during the night, you may suffer from sleep apnea. These gaps in breathing can last anywhere from 10 seconds to a minute, and you may have a snoring problem, too. Yet you may not be aware anything is wrong. What you will realize is how sleepy you are during the day. Sleep apnea increases your risk of heart disease, depression, headaches, and memory loss, so you should see your doctor. The first thing she'll tell you to do is lose weight if you're overweight. Other options include sleeping on your side, mouth appliances, surgery, injections, palate implants, and tongue and throat exercises.

Put out the flames of GERD. Gastroesophageal reflux disease — or the backup of stomach acid into your esophagus — is uncomfortable anytime of day, but nighttime heartburn can be agony. It can hit you at any age and doesn't care if you are male, female, fat, or thin. While a daily dose of antacid may be your only salvation, you can help put out the fire by adjusting your diet and lifestyle.

- Eat small meals and avoid eating anything heavy just before bedtime.

- Eliminate spicy, fatty, and acidic foods, like onions, tomatoes, and citrus.

- Cut down on coffee and alcohol.

- Raise the head of your bed so you're not lying flat at night.

- Find out if any medicines could be causing your reflux.

Calm restless legs for a quieter night. A night spent with twitching, tingling, achy legs is hard to sleep through. Not surprisingly, the symptoms of restless legs syndrome (RLS) are always worse when you're still and usually develop between 10 p.m. and 4 a.m. Certain forms of RLS run in families. Sometimes it's a problem with the nervous system. And sometimes it's a result of certain medical conditions, medications, or environmental factors. All you really want to know is how to make it stop.

- Talk to your doctor about potential causes. She may prescribe new medications or change existing ones.

- Try hot baths or cold compresses.

- Get some exercise each day.

- Stretch your calves or massage your legs before bed.

- Change your sleep schedule so you sleep later into the morning.

- Avoid caffeine and alcohol.

Dangers of daytime drowsiness

It's a myth that you need less sleep the older you get. Your body still requires about eight hours of shuteye to restore itself at night, but that's harder to get as you age. What's different is your overall health, the amount and kind of medications you may be taking, your activity level, and your sleep pattern. The result of all this daytime drowsiness is a higher risk of accidents, both in the car and out. The National Highway Traffic Safety Administration says more than 100,000 crashes a year are due to groggy drivers. And a study of seniors who slept less than six hours a night found they were three times more likely to fall numerous times in the follow-up year.

Sleep strategies

stick to a schedule • avoid naps • don't exercise at bedtime • take a hot bath • keep your bedroom cool • don't watch the clock

Sleep does as much good for your brain as it does for your body. Cut back on your sleep by even an hour or two, and you'll have trouble doing complicated projects or making big decisions. Getting the rest and relaxation you need is not a luxury — it's a necessity for long-term health.

Dream away your forgetfulness. Fascinating new research shows how getting enough sleep helps your brain work better. Natural sleep restores your body and your mind. It gives you enough dreaming time, or REM sleep, to sustain learning, memory, and mood. If you don't get enough sleep, you're more likely to make mistakes, suffer from depression and irritability, and have trouble learning new things and remembering old ones.

Researchers studied people who were either well rested or sleep deprived, asking them to do simple tasks while brain-imaging scans measured blood flow in the brain. The scans, called functional MRIs, showed lapses in certain areas of the brains of sleep-deprived people, even while they worked hard to complete the tasks.

This study showed how just one night of lost sleep can bring on what seems like a "power failure" in your brain. You'll have mental lapses and feel like you're in a fuzzy state between sleeping and waking.

Snooze your way to less stress. Not getting enough sleep also puts your body under stress. This can trigger the release of too much adrenaline, cortisol, and other stress hormones. These hormones help protect you in times of danger, but too much can keep your blood pressure from naturally falling during sleep, raising your risk of heart disease.

And it's a vicious cycle. When you're under stress, you may have more trouble getting the sleep you need. A National Sleep Foundation poll found nearly half of Americans surveyed had trouble with insomnia right after the terrorist attacks on September 11, 2001.

Sleep away belly fat. Sleep deprivation can make you gain weight — and it's not all about that leftover apple pie you wolf down in the middle of the night. Lack of sleep can alter your hunger hormones, giving you a lower level of leptin, which tells you you're full, and a higher level of ghrelin, which signals hunger.

These off-kilter hormones may lead you to eat more than you need. In fact, research shows lack of sleep is related to higher rates of metabolic syndrome — excess belly fat, high cholesterol, trouble controlling your blood sugar, and high blood pressure, which increases your risk of heart disease, stroke, and diabetes.

You can push back against memory-robbing problems with good sleep. Try these six super-simple steps to get the perfect night's sleep that will stop stress and boost your brain power at the same time.

6 sleep strategies that keep you sharp

Establish a regular bedtime routine. Go to bed at roughly the same time every night and wake up at the same time every morning. You may be tempted to sleep in on the weekends. Resist the temptation and stick to a schedule. Also plan some time for a relaxing activity before bedtime, like reading or listening to music, to help you wind down. But avoid pursuits like watching television or working on the computer just before bed. The lights from their bright screens can leave you too pumped up to get to sleep.

Avoid naps. You may think a midafternoon siesta will help you make it to bedtime, but a nap may do more harm than good. Sleeping during the day — especially in the late afternoon — can disrupt your body's natural sleep cycle and make it harder to fall asleep at night.

Don't exercise too close to bedtime. Physical activity during the day is a great way to get your body ready for sleep at night. One study found that exercise works as well for inducing sleep as taking a benzodiazepine prescription sleeping pill. Practicing yoga is especially good, because it involves meditation, deep breathing, and movements focusing on stretching and balance.

But don't exercise several hours before bed. Doing this can rev up your body and your mind, making it hard to relax in preparation for sleep.

Enjoy a hot bath. Take it about one or two hours before bed. Besides being relaxing, a bath will alter your body's core temperature, making it easier to fall asleep and sleep continuously through the night. Your body temperature tends to drop after you get out of a hot bath, mimicking what happens as your body gets ready for sleep.

Don't lie in bed stewing over your problems or that long to-do list. Keep a notebook and pen by your bed so you can write down whatever worry is keeping your brain active. Then tell yourself the problem is down on paper and off your mind. You'll be able to relax and fall asleep.

Keep your bedroom cool. Experts say the ideal temperature for sleep is 60 to 72 degrees Fahrenheit. Lowering your body's temperature can bring on sleep, so it makes sense to aim for a feeling of coolness in the bedroom.

If menopause is making you wake up overheated in the middle of the night, pay attention to your bed coverings. If you're using a big quilt, try just a sheet instead. Also consider clothing made to keep you cool, like pajamas made from bamboo, which has great wicking ability. You may also want to turn on a fan in the room to boost air circulation, or even set the fan to blow across a pan of ice cubes to keep you cool.

Don't watch the clock. Obsessing over the time makes it harder to sleep. Having a bad attitude about your sleeplessness makes it worse. If you find yourself awake in the middle of the night, try to avoid these repeated negative thoughts — "I'm not getting enough sleep, so I'll feel terrible tomorrow," "I hate it when I can't sleep," and "I'm angry about my insomnia."

Instead, change the way you think about your wakefulness, and trade those negative thoughts for positive ones — "I've had sleepless nights before, and I made it through just fine," "I'm probably getting some rest just lying here quietly," or "It's nice and quiet this time of the night." These positive thoughts will help you relax more than counting the hours until your alarm will sound.

Reset your sleep clock to reclaim lost memories

"For everything there is a season, a time for every activity under heaven." There's a time to sleep and a time to be awake. Circadian rhythm, sometimes called your biological clock, tells your body to sleep when it's dark and be awake when it's light. Get a little time in the sun, and you can improve your sleep and reclaim lost memories.

Circadian rhythm is controlled by the natural cycle of darkness and light. When less light enters your eyes, that's a signal for the pineal gland in your brain to start releasing melatonin, a hormone important for sleep. Circadian rhythm also controls patterns of eating, digestion, alertness, body temperature, and even blood pressure highs and lows.

Anything that interferes with how your body experiences the natural cycle of light and dark — including spending too much time indoors or bright artificial light in the evening — can hamper your sleep. Let your body know what time it is during the day, and you'll sleep better at night. Spend about 30 minutes in the sun every day to reset your body's clock. Go for a walk, play a game of tennis, or weed your garden and get a dose of bright sunshine.

Sleeping well may also help boost your memory and sharpen your mind. While you're sleeping, your brain is busy organizing memories and storing them more efficiently, making them more permanent. During sleep you also strengthen the connections between brain cells and among different parts of your brain. This keeps your memories, skills, and other knowledge from eroding over time.

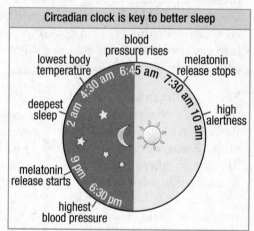

Circadian clock is key to better sleep

blood pressure rises

lowest body temperature

melatonin release stops

deepest sleep

high alertness

melatonin release starts

highest blood pressure

2 am 4:30 am 6:45 am 7:30 am 10 am 6:30 pm 9 pm

High-tech way to get some shut-eye

Research shows wearing special glasses or using special light bulbs can reset your biological clock to improve sleep.

Blocking light on the blue end of the spectrum a few hours before bedtime lets melatonin release begin early. Typically, melatonin starts to be released once you enter darkness. But when blue light is blocked from entering your eyes, you may be able to get to sleep earlier.

You can buy special blue-blocking glasses for as little as $40, or try special coated light bulbs that block blue lightwaves for about $5. See *www.lowbluelights.com* to buy these products from the company started by the researchers who developed this trick.

Sidestep sleeping pill dangers

A 24-year-old Scottish man taking prescription sleeping pills sleepwalked through an open window, becoming paralyzed from the accident. Odd behaviors like sleepwalking, sleep driving, and even sleep shoplifting can happen when you take some drugs to help you sleep. Many also can cause short-term memory problems or confusion.

Sleeping pills can help you get the rest you need when you suffer from a short-term problem that robs you of sleep, like pain or other stressful situation. But you shouldn't take these drugs longer than a few days or weeks. Some are habit-forming. And with some, you will need a higher and higher dose to keep working.

And there's more. Even when a sleeping pill works, you may wake up groggy the next day or suffer from rebound insomnia — trouble sleeping the following night that's even worse than your original problem. Sleep drugs can have serious interactions with other drugs or alcohol, and some can lead to physical problems like high blood pressure, dizziness, weakness, and nausea.

> Skip the nightcap. Drinking alcohol may seem like an ideal way to wind down in the evening. But if you have a drink just before bedtime, the alcohol clears your system a few hours later — when you'd rather be sleeping. This causes you to wake up in the middle of the night. Then it can be hard to get back to sleep.

Even more scary, some common sedatives, including zolpidem (Ambien), zaleplon (Sonata), and eszopiclone (Lunesta), can lead to delirium, which comes on suddenly and can cause changes in your vision, hearing, or thinking.

Talk to your doctor about the dangers if you're considering taking sleeping pills. She may offer suggestions about alternative remedies.

Socialization

volunteering • gathering with friends • attending church • working part-time • mentoring young people • joining a book club

The brain is proof you can still teach an old dog new tricks. Healthy brains are able to learn, even in old age. One way to do that, experts say, is to engage in stimulating activities, like socializing.

Harvard researchers found memory declined twice as fast in people who were the least socially active, compared to those who were the most. Did these social butterflies party all night to protect their memories? No. They were simply more likely to be married, to volunteer, or to stay in touch with family and neighbors.

Stress less. Psychological stress can lead to a breakdown in the hippocampus, the part of your brain linked to memory and emotion. People who are more prone to stress or have a harder time coping with it face a higher risk of Alzheimer's disease (AD) — unless they stay socially active. Having friends and a supportive network of people around you can lower your stress levels and help you cope better.

Beat the blues. Social circles fight depression, too, a disease that nearly doubles your risk of dementia, including AD. Depression affects your brain in three main ways.

- People suffering from depression have lower levels of a substance that keeps the brain flexible and enables it to make and store memories.

- Episodes of depression may lead your body to secrete compounds toxic to brain cells, eventually shrinking the hippocampus.

- Depression and the strain of it can cause chronic inflammation in your body, which in turn contributes to dementia, particularly AD.

Luckily, the same things that make you feel good, like laughing with friends or helping a neighbor, can help you beat the blues and guard your memory.

Beef up your brain. Social gatherings give your brain a workout, thanks to the skills needed to remember names and engage in conversation. Mingling may help lower blood pressure and improve other health problems linked to memory and brain health, too.

Social activities that make you think, like mentoring a child, pack a double punch. They boost your own problem-solving skills while adding meaning to your life, which makes them that much more rewarding. Plus, they help your brain grow new cells and repair itself when things go wrong, two keys in preventing Alzheimer's and other forms of dementia.

Banish loneliness. Loneliness itself can take a toll on your body. Feeling disconnected from others raises your risk for dementia. Experts say social activities that keep these feelings at bay may benefit your brain in their own way.

4 ways to socialize that keep you sharp

Consider old-time religion. Drawing closer to God could be good for your brain. Many studies link religious activities to better brain function.

- Older Mexican Americans who attended church at least monthly declined more slowly than people who didn't go to church.

- In Connecticut, people who went to church at least once a week were less likely to develop mental decline over the next three years.

Getting involved could be especially good if you suffer from depression, which is closely tied to mental decline. Yet another study showed attending church at least once a month protected people's brains, even if they suffered from depression.

Taking part in a religious community involves socializing with others, a known antidote to the blues. And it can give you hope and a sense of meaning, which lessens the severity of depression.

A loved one with dementia may eventually need more care than you can give them at home. That's when assisted living facilities or nursing homes become an option. Just make sure the one you choose offers plenty of creative and well-planned social activities for the residents. Research suggests care homes often don't provide enough companionship or daytime activities. That lack can worsen anxiety and depression in people with dementia.

The social support and interaction you get from church may also lower your levels of the hormone cortisol. Depressed people have higher levels than normal, and high cortisol may harm mental function. By reducing cortisol, church attendance may dampen depression's impact on the brain.

The fellowship you gain may even provide a buffer against the harmful effects of stress. Research suggests the emotional support from fellow church members helps prevent problems, like money worries, from harming your health. Building a closer relationship with God, on the other hand, can help you feel more optimistic and hopeful, which enables you to cope better with stressful events and illnesses.

Find a purpose. Simply having a sense of purpose in life protects against Alzheimer's disease (AD), mild cognitive impairment, and mental decline. Out of 900 older adults, those who reported having the greatest sense of purpose:

- were 2.4 times less likely to develop AD.

- were less likely to develop mild cognitive impairment with age.

- declined more slowly over seven years than people with a low sense of purpose.

You don't have to be born with one. It's something you can develop. Get involved in causes you think matter. Participate in activities that are personally meaningful to you. Do the things in your life with intention, rather than aimlessly. Set goals, and act with those goals in mind.

Say 'no' to retirement. Seniors who either keep working after retirement age or begin volunteering score significantly better on thinking tests, are less depressed, and enjoy greater mental well-being and satisfaction with life.

Experts point to the interaction and engagement you get from these activities. You meet people and expand your social network, a key to healthy aging. A job or volunteer work can also give life a sense of meaning that keeps you going. Plus, it gives your brain a workout and the opportunity to learn new things. In fact, older retirees gain more brain benefits from continuing to work than younger ones.

Become a mentor. Mentoring a child could be the secret to staying young in both the heart and mind. Eight senior women at high risk for mental decline began volunteering their time at local elementary schools through a program called Experience Corps. They spent 15 hours each week helping children improve their reading and library skills.

The seniors helped themselves at least as much as they did the kids. These women didn't just maintain their brain health. They improved it, beefing up the areas involved in planning, problem solving, and reasoning skills. These are the same areas that keep you independent and functional, yet they are especially prone to fail with age.

Experts say programs like Experience Corps could reverse the age-related loss of brain power. To find an Experience Corps program near you, call the organization at 202-478-6190 or visit *experiencecorps.org* on the Internet.

You can volunteer at a soup kitchen or donate money to charity. No matter how you give of yourself, you'll get something back in health benefits.

Social activities can keep your mind sharp, but choosing charitable and compassionate ways of connecting with people will help you live longer, too. Lending a helping hand to others can even give you more energy, ease aches and pains, and make you feel stronger, calmer, and better about yourself.

Trade solo for social for more brainpower

Try doing typically solo activities with a group to keep your mind keen. It's easy to turn activities like these into social events.

taking walks	Start a walking club with friends or neighbors.
gardening	Join a community garden where you can teach others how to grow flowers, fruits, and vegetables.
watching television	Catch your favorite show with friends, and take turns hosting the weekly viewing party.
reading	Look for a local book club that focuses on genres you like.
cooking	Start a monthly recipe swap with your friends, where you try out new dishes and share the recipes.
handy work	Volunteer your skills for a good cause with a group like Habitat for Humanity.

4 mental mistakes to avoid now

Mental decline is not a normal part of aging. Steer clear of these traps to keep your brain sharp into the future.

Letting stress get to you. People who are easily stressed out are more likely to develop depression and Alzheimer's disease. Maintaining an active social life may help lessen this risk.

Negative thinking. Pessimism can be a symptom of depression, a condition that boosts your risk of dementia. Negativity is contagious, so surround yourself with positive people. Make a list every day of the good things that happened, and stop yourself when you start having negative thoughts. See your doctor if you have trouble shaking the blues.

Not challenging your brain. Exercise your brain if you want it to last into your 90s. Mental challenges, such as crossword puzzles and music classes, build up your brain reserve, like putting money in a savings account. The bigger your reserve, the longer it will take for age to dull your thinking.

Going through life alone. No man, or woman, is an island, but behaving like one could lead to faster mental decline. An active social life — complete with friends, family, neighbors, and causes you care about — can challenge your mind, beat back depression, and reduce your risk of Alzheimer's disease and other types of dementia.

Soluble fiber

oats • barley • beans • peas • lentils • nuts
• seeds • citrus fruits • apples • bananas • pears
• strawberries • blueberries • carrots

Nolan Ryan could light up the radar gun with his blazing fastball. He struck out a whopping 5,714 batters and won 324 games during his career. On the other hand, Phil Niekro relied on a slow, baffling knuckle ball to record 3,342 strikeouts and 318 wins. Both pitchers are in the Baseball Hall of Fame.

Like these two baseball legends, the two main types of fiber — soluble and insoluble — employ different tactics to succeed. Insoluble fiber, like Ryan, uses speed. By zipping stool through your large intestine, insoluble fiber helps keep you regular. Learn more about the benefits of insoluble fiber in the *Insoluble fiber* chapter.

Soluble fiber, like Niekro, works by slowing things down. Also known as viscous fiber, soluble fiber binds with water to form a gel, which delays the emptying of your stomach and slows the movement of food through your small intestine.

Not only does this curb your appetite by making you feel fuller longer — it also helps lower your cholesterol and control your blood sugar and insulin levels.

Found in dried beans and peas, oats, barley, and citrus fruits, soluble fiber can be a boon to your brain because it shields your body from so many conditions that can harm it.

For example, oatmeal may just be the best breakfast food ever. As a good source of soluble fiber, oatmeal protects against weight gain and lowers cholesterol, high blood pressure, and type 2 diabetes. Read on to

1/3 cup uncooked oatmeal	1.4 g*
3/4 cup oat bran	2.2 g
1/2 cup black beans	2.4 g
1/2 cup kidney beans	2.8 g
1/2 cup brussels sprouts	2 g
1/2 cup asparagus	1.7 g
1 small orange	1.8 g
1 slice pumpernickel bread	1.2 g

* milligrams

discover how oatmeal and other sources of soluble fiber can help you strike out disease and win the battle against dementia.

5 ways soluble fiber keeps you sharp

Lowers cholesterol. This is soluble fiber's claim to fame — and with good reason. Several studies have demonstrated soluble fiber's ability to bring down cholesterol levels.

High cholesterol doesn't just put you at high risk for atherosclerosis, heart attack, and stroke — it also puts your brain in danger. That's because oxygen- and nutrient-rich blood has trouble making its way through stiff, narrow — or completely blocked — arteries and reaching your brain. When brain cells die from lack of oxygen or because of a clot-induced stroke, you can develop vascular dementia, the second most common form of dementia after Alzheimer's disease.

In one study of almost 10,000 people, those in their 40s with high cholesterol increased their risk of Alzheimer's disease later in life by

66 percent. Even if their levels were only borderline high, they increased their risk by 52 percent. Add some soluble fiber to your diet, and bring that risk down.

Six grams a day of concentrated oat beta-glucan, a soluble fiber, significantly lowered total and harmful LDL cholesterol in one six-week study. Dutch researchers found that beta-glucan, when added to fruit drinks, lowers cholesterol by increasing bile acid secretion and decreasing cholesterol absorption.

Psyllium, another soluble fiber, also works. In one study, taking 15 grams of psyllium along with 10 milligrams (mg) of simvastatin was just as effective at lowering cholesterol as a 20-mg dose of simvastatin. A Spanish study showed that psyllium husk, rich in soluble fiber, boosted good HDL cholesterol and helped lower other heart disease risk factors better than psyllium seeds, which contain insoluble fiber.

But you don't need to take supplements to reap the benefits of soluble fiber. Oatmeal and other foods rich in soluble fiber do the trick. A recent review of eight oat-based studies confirmed that oats helped lower LDL cholesterol by an average of 5 percent.

Canadian researchers found that a diet consisting of proven cholesterol-lowering foods — including soluble fiber from oats,

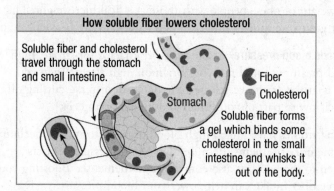

How soluble fiber lowers cholesterol

Soluble fiber and cholesterol travel through the stomach and small intestine.

Fiber

Cholesterol

Stomach

Soluble fiber forms a gel which binds some cholesterol in the small intestine and whisks it out of the body.

barley, psyllium, okra, and eggplant — worked just as well as a statin to lower cholesterol. Other studies have found positive effects for pinto beans and nuts. Aim for at least 3 grams of soluble fiber a day to lower cholesterol.

Protects against weight gain. Body fat — especially belly fat — takes a heavy toll on your brain. If you're carrying too many pounds, you're also lugging around a 42 percent higher risk of dementia compared to someone at a healthier weight. If that extra weight sits mostly around your middle, you've almost tripled the likelihood you'll develop dementia.

The deadly trio of obesity, heart disease, and diabetes spells trouble for healthy blood flow and affects how you're able to think in so many ways. Excess weight is tangled up with blood pressure, cholesterol, and blood sugar, so it's almost impossible to fix any of these problems without controlling your weight.

Shrink belly fat faster with whole grains like oatmeal. A recent astounding study proves that a diet rich in whole grains, including oatmeal, helps you lose weight and reduce abdominal fat. Oatmeal, known as a folksy cure for itchy skin, provides soluble fiber and also serves as a high-volume, low-energy density food that fills you up without adding too many calories.

University of Southern California researchers compared the diets of overweight or obese people with those at a healthier weight. The latter group ate much more fiber and fruit than the heavier group.

Reduces blood pressure. As the major risk factor for stroke, high blood pressure should put your brain on high alert. When you have a stroke, blood vessels become blocked or burst, cutting off blood flow to part of your brain and killing brain cells.

Several studies have linked high blood pressure to mental decline and memory problems. Because high blood pressure restricts oxygen to the brain, it also contributes to dementia. Boosting your soluble fiber intake can help lower your blood pressure.

In one study, researchers found that whole grains — including barley, a source of soluble fiber — helped lower blood pressure. No wonder whole grains are a key component of the Dietary Approaches to Stop Hypertension (DASH) diet.

Most studies of oat products, like oatmeal, show a positive effect on blood pressure. An older Australian study found that drinking a mixture of psyllium and soy protein helped lower blood pressure for people with high blood pressure.

Guards against diabetes. Keeping your blood sugar in check helps keep your brain working. Besides upping your risk for a heart attack or stroke, diabetes also affects how well you think and remember. If glucose doesn't reach your brain cells, they don't have enough energy to function properly. This can lead to a vicious cycle of decline. When your thinking is impaired, you may not take your diabetes medication properly, eat right, or remember to exercise. Your diabetes gets worse, which further impacts your mental abilities.

New research finds that both diabetes and Alzheimer's disease are affected by lack of insulin. Men who didn't produce the right amount of insulin at age 50 were at a significantly greater risk of developing Alzheimer's disease and other types of dementia later on. People with diabetes also have more than a 50 percent higher risk of depression.

That morning cup of coffee gives you more than a jolt of caffeine — it also provides a surprising dose of soluble fiber. Spanish researchers found that coffee contains more soluble fiber than wine or orange juice. Instant coffee gives you the most soluble fiber at 1.8 grams per cup, while espresso (1.5 grams) and filtered coffee (1.1 grams) contain a little less.

Luckily, adding soluble fiber to your diet can help. In one small study, a moderate amount of beta-glucan helped lower both the glucose and insulin responses for over-weight and healthy weight women. The viscosity, or stickiness, of the soluble fiber likely delays or reduces the absorption of carbohydrates from the gut.

An older study found that boosting soluble fiber intake — through foods like oatmeal, oat bran, granola, cantaloupe, grapefruit, orange, papaya, raisins, lima beans, okra, sweet potato, winter squash, and zucchini — improved glycemic control and lowered cholesterol in people with diabetes. People in the study ate 25 grams of soluble fiber and 25 grams of insoluble fiber each day.

Insoluble fiber gets most of the credit for fiber's beneficial effect on your digestive tract. But recent studies suggest that soluble fiber may actually provide more relief for certain digestive disorders, such as irritable bowel syndrome (IBS) and Crohn's disease. If you have IBS, consider switching from bran to psyllium.

Soluble fiber supplements also worked to lower LDL cholesterol and boost HDL cholesterol in people with diabetes.

Stops inflammation. Your body needs occasional inflammation to fight off bacteria and viruses. But chronic inflammation interferes with certain processes within your body and destroys tissues. Eventually, this damage puts you at risk of developing some very serious conditions, like diabetes, heart disease, Alzheimer's disease, arthritis, and cancer.

A recent University of Illinois study found that soluble fiber, in the form of citrus pectin, boosted the immune system of mice. Researchers noted that soluble fiber changed the nature of immune cells from pro-inflammatory to anti-inflammatory, thanks to an increase in an anti-inflammatory protein called interleukin-4.

One marker of inflammation is a protein called C-reactive protein (CRP). If your CRP levels remain high for too long, experts think your risk of heart disease, stroke, high blood pressure, diabetes, and insulin resistance go up. CRP is also associated with thinking and memory problems, as well as dementia.

In one study, people whose diet contained the most soluble fiber lowered their risk for elevated CRP levels by 61 percent compared to those who ate the least.

Make the most of oats

Starting your day with a hot bowl of oatmeal is an easy — and tasty — way to get more soluble fiber into your diet. But you can also sprinkle some oats into your pancake batter to add a healthy bit of texture.

Of course, oats aren't just for breakfast. You can find some creative yet simple strategies to slip more oats into your diet throughout the day. For example, oats can act as a binder when you make hamburgers or meatloaf. You can also use oats as part of a homemade granola or as a breading for chicken pieces.

Little-known drug interaction

Do not take your medications and fiber supplements at the same time. Otherwise, you may not be getting all the medication you need. That's because your body doesn't absorb or digest fiber, and the drugs can get swept out of your body along with the fiber.

Fiber supplements, such as psyllium, guar gum, and pectin, may reduce or slow the absorption of certain medications, including blood-thinning drugs like warfarin, anti-clotting drugs like Plavix, and cholesterol-lowering drugs like Crestor and lovastatin. Even Tylenol and penicillin may be affected. Your best bet is to play it safe. Take any medication about two hours before or after you take your fiber supplements.

But that doesn't mean you need to worry about fiber from foods interacting with your drugs. Even high-fiber meals are OK. The risk applies only to fiber supplements.

Pectin is a soluble fiber often added to jellies and jams as a thickening agent. Crab apple contains natural pectin so this recipe doesn't require pectin as a separate ingredient. Try this fiber-rich, no-fat spread on whole-grain bread for a delicious and nutritious treat.

Fiber-rich crabapple jelly

8 cups fresh crab apples

3 cups granulated sugar

1 cinnamon stick

Remove stems and blossoms from the crab apples. Cut into quarters and put them in a large pan of water. Make sure the water covers the crab apples, but not so much that they float.

Bring water to a boil and then turn down to simmer. Add the cinnamon stick to the water. Simmer for 15 minutes or until apples are soft.

Strain the apples and juice through two or three layers of cheesecloth until you have 4 cups of clear juice. Discard the pulp.

Pour the juice back into the pan. Simmer for 10 minutes.

Skim off foam. Stir in sugar until dissolved. Cook on low boil until the temperature reaches 220 to 222 degrees.

Pour into small canning jars, leaving 1/4-inch space at the top. Process in hot water bath to seal.

The jelly may take several days to set — so be patient.

Makes about 6 8-oz. jars

Spices

sage • rosemary • chamomile

You may be surprised at what you don't know about aromatic spices like sage, rosemary, and chamomile. These ancient seasonings not only lend fabulous flavors to cooking, they may help protect your health.

Sage has been used as a seasoning and medicine for centuries. In fact, experts are still trying to identify all the healthy antioxidants it contains. Over 500 species of sage exist, but garden sage *(salvia officinalis)* and Spanish sage *(salvia lavandulifolia)* may hold the most promise for your brain and memory.

The rosemary plant is a fragrant evergreen shrub. Rosemary often grows near the sea, which may be why its botanical name, *Rosmarinus*, means "dew of the sea." This seemingly simple plant is packed with powerful antioxidants. Just smelling this spice may have positive effects on your health, aromatherapy studies suggest. But you may benefit from eating rosemary, too.

Chamomile may look like a roadside daisy, but it is so much more. The German nickname for chamomile is "alles zustraut" meaning "capable of anything."

Although the Germans are only talking about one kind of chamomile, you'll actually find two kinds of chamomile used for health. German chamomile *(Matricaria recutita)* grows about 18 inches high and is popular in the United States and central Europe. Roman chamomile *(Anthemis nobilis* or *Chamaemelum nobile)* is a low-growing chamomile popular in the United Kingdom.

3 spices that keep you sharp

Sage. You can choose from many natural and even fun solutions to help you avoid Alzheimer's and fight brain aging. For example, keeping your brain healthy for the long term can be almost as simple as going to your garden, or the fresh produce aisle, and choosing something delicious. Studies even suggest one type of incredible plant — sage — may be a prime pick for lasting brainpower.

Normally, your brain uses a compound called acetylcholine to perform tasks that create your short-term memory. These tasks are called cholinergic function. In people with Alzheimer's disease, cholinergic function starts failing. Fortunately, persuading your brain to add more acetylcholine seems to help, and sage may have the power to do that.

In a small study, people with mild-to-moderate Alzheimer's disease who took a sage extract for four months scored better on tests of mental abilities than people who took a placebo. What's more, sage is not just good for people with Alzheimer's. Research has also linked sage to improvements in the memory and mental abilities of healthy adults.

Although most studies have used concentrated sources of sage, such as an extract or essential oil, reports also suggest people can get results from the equivalent of 1 1/2 teaspoons of garden sage a day. Still, as few as 12 drops of sage essential oil or tinctures may cause seizures if taken internally. Don't try them without guidance from your doctor.

One box of chamomile tea bags is labeled German chamomile, while the other is labeled Roman chamomile. Which should you choose? German chamomile and Roman chamomile have similar effects, but German chamomile tastes sweeter and may pack slightly more healing power. German chamomile is also better researched and more widely used.

On the other hand, if you want to grow sage in your garden, there are hundreds of varieties to choose from. Just keep in mind that two varieties are known for their success in studies, garden sage *(salvia officinalis)* and Spanish sage *(salvia lavandulifolia)*.

Rosemary. The ancient Greeks used rosemary to chase away evil spirits and poor health. Today, modern research suggests they may have had the right idea. Dangerous free radicals created by natural body processes contribute to Alzheimer's disease, strokes, and even normal brain aging.

Not surprisingly, rosemary contains a powerful antioxidant called carnosic acid that may help neutralize free radicals. Recent research suggests carnosic acid accumulates in brain cells, so it may stop free radical damage before it starts.

What's more, carnosic acid may help prevent the brain artery blockages that lead to strokes. That is good news because a stroke automatically raises your risk of Alzheimer's disease.

Research also suggests rosemary may inhibit an enzyme that interferes with acetylcholine, an important chemical messenger in your brain.

Chamomile. This delicate, flowering plant may help you fight two health issues that affect your brain, insomnia and high blood sugar.

- Insomnia. Sleep problems lead to sluggish reaction times, fuzzier thinking, inability to make decisions, and difficulty processing information. During sleep, memories are strengthened and integrated into the part of your brain responsible for forming new memories and storing long-term ones. It's no wonder research suggests sleep problems may affect your memory, too. A study of heart surgery patients accidentally discovered that chamomile tea might help promote sleep. Chamomile contains a compound called apigenin that seems to act as a mild sedative to help you snooze. Chamomile may also ease anxiety. Although more research is needed, experts suggest steeping a heaping teaspoon of dried chamomile flowers in hot water for 10 minutes to make a delicious tea. Drink up to three cups of this tea a day, and you may find it not only helps you sleep, it also improves your memory and thinking.

- High blood sugar. An animal study found that drinking chamomile tea with meals may help keep blood sugar down. Of course, animals don't always have the same reaction as humans, so more research is needed. But drinking chamomile tea is harmless for most people and taking steps to control your blood sugar may help prevent diabetes or its complications. On top of that, avoiding diabetes may also help protect your brain from Alzheimer's disease.

Grow your own spices

There's a great way to get cheaper, fresher spices — just pick chamomile, rosemary, and sage right from your garden. Here's how to start.

Chamomile. To grow either Roman or German chamomile:

- Buy seeds after the last spring frost.

- Sprinkle the seeds on moist soil in a sunny spot and water regularly.

- After a couple of weeks, plant the seedlings in the ground 18 inches apart.

- Harvest flowers when they reach peak bloom.

Rosemary. To grow rosemary:

- Buy a started rosemary plant instead of seeds.

- In a mild winter area, pick a sunny spot and plant your rosemary so it sits at the same depth in the ground as it did in the pot.

- Where winter temperatures fall below 25 degrees, plant rosemary in a container after the last frost. Bring it indoors for the winter when temperatures drop below freezing. Keep the plant in a south-facing window and water every time it becomes fully dry.

Sage. To grow sage:

- Plant newly bought seeds or seedlings in a sunny spot after the last frost.

- Space plants 30 inches apart and water regularly.

- Harvest lightly the first year and stop harvesting in early autumn to prepare the plant for winter.

And remember, avoid using sprays or pesticides on these plants. After all, you are going to eat them.

To get more sage in your diet, add chopped or whole sage leaves to these favorites:

- stuffing
- cornbread recipes
- pizza
- asparagus
- poultry and meat

- vegetable soups
- macaroni and cheese
- bread and biscuit recipes
- winter squash
- tomato-based sauces

Beware the dark side of spices

Sage, rosemary, and chamomile are generally regarded as safe when used as spices, but here are several reasons why you may prefer to play it safe and talk to your doctor before using them.

- Some spices may interact with certain medications or influence the results of blood and lab tests.

- Stay away from chamomile if you have allergies to onions, celery, or any members of the aster family, including asters, ragweed, sunflowers, and chrysanthemums. If you are allergic to any of these, you are more likely to be allergic to chamomile, too.

- Talk to your doctor before using rosemary if you take lithium or have concerns about low iron levels. Rosemary may decrease your ability to absorb iron and may lead to a toxic drug interaction with lithium.

Stress

increased heart rate • rapid breathing • dry mouth • cold sweat • stomach problems • headache • sleep problems • impaired memory

Stress can come in handy. In times of danger, it prepares your body for action. An immediate threat, such as a charging rhinoceros, triggers the release of the stress hormone cortisol as well as the neurotransmitters dopamine, norepinephrine, and epinephrine — known collectively as catecholamines.

During this "fight or flight" response, your heart rate and blood pressure go up, your blood flow increases, your breathing speeds up, and your immune system gears up to deal with potential injuries. When the threat passes, everything returns to normal.

Or at least it should. The problem is that everyday pressures — including financial worries, relationship issues, health problems, job demands, and traffic jams — can trigger the same response, without much time to recover. This chronic stress takes its toll on both your physical and mental health.

Chronic stress has been linked to high blood pressure, heart disease, and stroke. It also weakens your immune system, so you heal more slowly and get sick more often.

But stress really strikes your brain. When you have trouble adapting to stress, it can lead to

> Your nose knows how to relieve stress. Just try aroma-therapy. Scents such as green apple, cucumber, lavender, and rosemary can help you relax. Oranges, grapes, mangos, lemons, and basil may also help, thanks to a floral scented compound called linalool.

depression or anxiety. Scientists say, over time, stress and depression damage brain cells. A 20-year University of Pittsburgh study found that chronic life stress led to a decrease in the volume of the hippocampus, a brain region essential for learning and memory.

Other studies have linked high levels of stress hormones to worse memory, focus, and problem-solving skills. That makes sense, because a barrage of stress hormones can shrink brain cells and disrupt connections between them.

Stress can be quite a menace. It harms your heart, shrinks your brain, and attacks your immune system — and you probably experience it every day. But you can fight it without drugs.

However, if your stress becomes unmanageable, you may want to seek professional help. But there are several simple, natural ways to prevent or treat stress.

6 tactics to fight stress

Sweat it out. Exercise does wonders for stress. Not only does it distract you from your troubles, it also reduces stress's harmful effects on your blood pressure and heart. One study found that moderate to vigorous exercise was second only to prescription medication for reducing anxiety. Go for a brisk walk, swim laps, or try tai chi or yoga, which include stress-relieving benefits like breathing and muscle relaxation.

Sleep it off. Make sure you get enough sleep. At night, your blood pressure and cortisol levels should go down — but that doesn't happen when you're sleep deprived. Operating on little sleep also affects your mood and ability to make decisions. It may be tough to get quality sleep when you're stressed, but not getting enough sleep just makes things worse. Practice good sleep hygiene to get your 40 winks.

Laugh out loud. Calm stress, boost your mood, and feel better about the future with one proven treatment that doesn't require a doctor. It doesn't even cost money. Sometimes, laughter really is the best medicine. It's important to keep your sense of humor, especially during stressful times.

Laughter lowers cortisol and epinephrine levels and stimulates your immune system, counteracting the damages of stress. It can also relax your blood vessels and increase blood flow. Just anticipating laughter can have beneficial effects. Even if you're not in the jolliest of moods, forcing yourself to laugh can improve it. Watch a funny movie or talk to a humorous friend to boost your spirits and lower your stress.

Dark chocolate may be a sweet way to stymie stress. In a recent study, highly stressed people who ate 1.4 ounces of dark chocolate a day for two weeks reduced their levels of the stress hormones cortisol and the catecholamines. Enjoy dark chocolate in moderation, and you may lighten your worries.

Interestingly, crying can also help. You may feel less angry and sad after crying because you're getting rid of chemicals that build up during stress.

Relax it away. There's not a one-size-fits-all answer for relieving stress, but you have several options. Listening to music, keeping a diary, going on vacation, getting a massage, trying acupuncture, or owning a pet may help.

You can also try the following relaxation techniques to find what works for you.

- Deep breathing exercises. Breathing slowly and deeply helps you wind down. Count to 10 as you inhale through your nose, then do the same on the exhale.

- Muscle relaxation. Lie down and tense then relax each muscle from head to toe. Focus on one area at a time. By the time you're done, you'll feel extremely relaxed.

- Biofeedback. This technique, which requires some equipment and training, teaches you to control breathing, heart rate, blood pressure, and other signs of stress.

Talk it out. Stress is hard enough to handle. Don't make it tougher by going it alone. Isolation makes stress worse. A recent study found that people prone to stress who are socially isolated are at greater risk for dementia. That's why it's so important to have people to talk to during tough times. Share your feelings with friends or family members — and make sure to listen to them, too. Volunteering, joining a club, or taking a class can help you meet new people. Reconnect with friends or relatives you haven't spoken to in a while. They'll probably be glad to hear from you.

Soothe it with supplements. Not every herb or dietary supplement delivers what it promises, but studies suggest some may help relieve stress and anxiety. Kava may work better than some prescription medicines used to treat anxiety, but it comes with the risk of liver damage. Valerian reduces sensations and symptoms of anxiety and also acts as a natural sleep aid. Other promising anxiety remedies include *Rhodiola rosea*, or golden root; *Bacopa monniera*, or Brahmi; and *Centella asiatica*, or gotu kola.

Coping strategies to avoid

There are many healthy ways to reduce stress — and many not-so-healthy ways. Don't turn to bad habits like smoking, drinking too much alcohol, and being a couch potato. And beware of poor food choices. When you're stressed, you tend to crave fatty, salty, or sugary foods. These coping strategies only add to your woes, putting you at higher risk for obesity, diabetes, cancer, and other health problems.

Don't believe the hype about quick, easy cures for stress. Supplements, including herbs, may seem safe and effective, but that's not always the case. You could waste your money or even risk dangerous side effects. Talk to your doctor before trying any supplements.

> Sip away your stress with a soothing cup of green tea. A recent Japanese study found that people who drank at least five cups of green tea a day were 20 percent less likely to develop mental stress than those who drank less than a cup a day.

Foods	Nutrient	How it fights stress in your body
bread, cereal, pasta	complex carbohydrates	boost serotonin levels in your brain to make you feel calmer
nuts, beans, meat	B vitamins	decrease cortisol response, improve sleep, help form key neurotransmitters
citrus fruit, strawberries	vitamin C	works with adrenal gland to limit production of the stress hormone cortisol
spinach, bran cereal, yogurt	magnesium	replenishes this key mineral, which is depleted by stress and anxiety
fish, walnuts, flaxseed	omega-3 fatty acids	keep cortisol and norepinephrine in check, reduce inflammation

Stroke

sudden weakness • vision loss • confusion
• loss of consciousness • speech problems
• severe headache • dizziness

The 100 billion neurons in your brain need massive amounts of blood to work properly. Or rather, they need the oxygen and nutrients your blood transports. In fact, about 20 percent of the total amount of blood your heart pumps out is sent to your brain. When this flow is interrupted, you suffer a stroke — and that's bad news for all those neurons. There are two basic kinds of stoke.

- Ischemic. An ischemic stroke occurs when a clot or other particle blocks an artery carrying blood to your brain. Without the life-giving nutrients, neurons begin to die. The extent of the damage depends on where the blockage is and how long it lasts. Most strokes are ischemic.

- Hemorrhagic. In a hemorrhagic stroke, also known as a bleeding stroke, an artery in your brain ruptures. Blood leaks into the surrounding brain tissue, or into the space between your brain and skull, damaging brain cells. Only about 20 percent of strokes are hemorrhagic.

Strokes can be damaging within minutes, catastrophic within hours. Depending on what part of your brain is affected and for how long, memory, motor skills, speech, behavior, and thought processes can all be impaired. You can also suffer less-obvious, long-term problems like depression and poor sleep.

The good news is you have some natural protection and recovery wired into your brain. If a major artery is blocked or tears, a ring of blood vessels at the base of your brain provides a substitute route for blood flow. It's sort of like a detour system in your brain.

And even though brain cells die during a stroke, other neurons gradually take over their jobs. In that way, many people who suffer a stroke recover some of the functions they initially lost.

Several health conditions, like high blood pressure and diabetes, make it more likely you'll suffer a stroke. But with some simple lifestyle changes, you can significantly cut your risk.

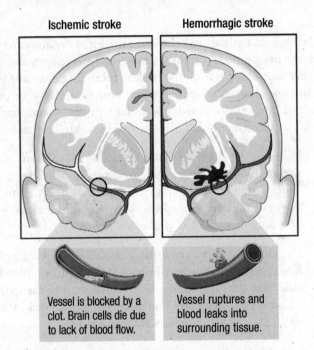

Ischemic stroke	Hemorrhagic stroke
Vessel is blocked by a clot. Brain cells die due to lack of blood flow.	Vessel ruptures and blood leaks into surrounding tissue.

Get savvy on stroke's danger signals

- sudden weakness or numbness on one side of your body
- sudden vision loss
- mental confusion or memory loss
- sudden loss of consciousness

- speech problems or difficulty understanding other people

- a sudden, severe headache

- unexplained dizziness or falls

- nausea and vomiting, especially when accompanied by any of the symptoms listed here

4 tactics to fight stroke

Beat blood pressure woes. If you have high blood pressure, your heart has to work extra hard to push blood through your circulatory system. Picture an old, stiff garden hose with a small nozzle on the end. Now imagine you've turned the water on high. Pressure inside the hose becomes enormous, and eventually you'll have a leak on your hands. That's just how high blood pressure weakens your artery walls. You, too, can spring a leak — a hemorrhagic stroke.

Damage to your artery walls from this high pressure can cause cholesterol and plaque to build up. These can eventually build up enough to clog the artery or break off causing a clot to form — resulting in an ischemic stroke. If you don't control your blood pressure, you're about five times more likely to have a stroke.

A transient ischemic attack or TIA is also known as a mini-stroke. You suffer many of the same symptoms as a full-blown stroke, but TIAs only last about five to 20 minutes and do not usually cause permanent damage. More than a third of the people who suffer a TIA eventually have an ischemic stroke. Think of a TIA as a warning. Call 911 immediately. If you have a stroke, the doctor might be able to give you a clot-busting drug called t-PA, which can greatly increase your odds of survival and recovery.

Keep blood pressure within bounds by exercising, maintaining a healthy weight, lowering your salt intake, and eating potassium-rich foods like beans, raisins, potatoes, and spinach.

Cope with climbing cholesterol. Cholesterol is a soft, waxy substance that travels through your bloodstream. It helps form cell membranes and other tissues, as well as some hormones. Your body needs cholesterol, but too much can clog your arteries. If enough accumulates, it can close off an artery completely, causing an ischemic stroke. Most vulnerable are the two big carotid arteries in your neck that supply blood to your brain. When one of these becomes narrowed, it's called carotid stenosis, and your risk of stroke multiplies by three. A clot or obstruction here can completely block blood flow to your brain.

Now a simple blood test can predict this silent killer. Approved by the FDA, the PLAC test measures an enzyme called lipoprotein-associated phospholipase A2 (Lp-PLA2), which is associated with inflammation in your arteries. If you have high levels of this enzyme, your risk of ischemic stroke is double that of someone with normal levels. Learn more about this test online at *www.plactest.com.*

Take charge of your cholesterol with a diet high in fiber from whole grains and beans, low in saturated fat from meat and dairy, and full of vegetables, fruits, and fish. Lose weight if you're carrying some extra pounds and do something active every day.

Put the rhythm back in your heart. Atrial fibrillation (AF), a type of irregular heartbeat, causes blood to collect in your heart. There it's likely to form clots, which frequently break free, travel to your brain, and cause a stroke. If you suffer from AF, your risk of stroke just went up by 500 percent. To keep your heart rhythm regular, you may need medication. If that's not successful, your doctor may prescribe a blood thinner to prevent blood clots from forming. If your doctor prescribes blood-thinning medication, talk with him about avoiding vitamin K-rich foods, which can cause your blood to clot.

You can check your pulse to see if it is even and consistent. An irregular pulse will fluctuate. Make an appointment to see your doctor if it's irregular.

Check your CRP. Whenever there is inflammation anywhere in your body, including your blood vessels, your liver produces a substance called C-reactive protein (CRP). Inflammation in your arteries and blood vessels creates what experts call "unstable lesions." These are damaged areas that are very likely to rupture and cause a stroke. That's why high CRP levels are now recognized as a stroke risk factor. Know what your CRP levels are. All it takes is a simple blood test. And work to bring inflammation down with vitamin C-rich foods, moderate exercise, weight control, and aspirin therapy.

Can you touch your toes? Go ahead and try it. Sit on the floor with your back against the wall and your legs stretched out in front of you. Now bend forward from the waist and reach. Researchers say this is a good way to measure not only how flexible your muscles are, but how flexible your arteries are.

Surprising stroke risks you should know

Three conditions increase your odds of suffering a stroke. Talk to your doctor about how to protect yourself if these apply to you.

- Diabetes. If you have diabetes, you probably have other health problems that make you vulnerable to stroke. In fact, your risk of ischemic stroke is three times higher than people without diabetes.

- Shingles. A case of shingles, the blistery rash triggered by the same virus that causes chickenpox, also multiplies the danger. You're four times more likely to have a stroke within a year if the rash is around your eyes or on your forehead.

- Gum disease. Severe gum disease can raise your risk of stroke by causing plaque to form in your carotid arteries, which supply blood to your brain. Reduced blood flow to your brain caused by a blockage can lead to an ischemic stroke.

Tai chi

prevents falls and brain injuries • reduces blood pressure
• wards off heart attacks and strokes • soothes stress
• promotes better sleep • fights memory loss
• lowers blood sugar

Visit a local park in China at dawn and you may see a group of people moving in synchronized slow motion, easing their way through a pattern of gentle, circular exercises that seem to flow from one to the next. This soothing exercise, called tai chi, was developed in China centuries ago.

To do tai chi, you learn to relax and breathe deeply while concentrating on learning a series of exercises or movements called forms. Some versions of tai chi have long forms with many movements, and some have short forms. Learning all the movements in a form can take awhile. If you are a first-timer, you may prefer a short-form version of tai chi.

Because tai chi includes relaxation, deep breathing, and concentration, you may hear it called "meditation in motion." But that does not mean tai chi is a religion you must follow. It's just a good way to relax, exercise, and improve your health. Anyone can benefit from this easy, slow-motion exercise, no matter their age. And the best part — some tai chi sessions take just 11 minutes a day.

6 ways tai chi keeps you sharp

Creates a no-fall zone. Tai chi can improve your balance, strength, and coordination, and these improvements help prevent falls. That's good news because falls are a leading cause of brain injury. A brain injury sets the stage for a slump in brain skills and raises your risk of Alzheimer's disease (AD) and other forms of dementia.

Helps you sleep better and longer. Six months of tai chi helped older adults with sleep problems sleep longer and more soundly. Older adults have more sleep disturbances because their sympathetic nervous system sends too many nighttime signals that promote rousing. The deep breathing, relaxation, and slow nature of tai chi may help ease this problem so it no longer interferes with sleep. That's important because even mild sleep loss can affect thinking and memory.

In one study, people who got only six hours of sleep a night reacted more slowly, couldn't think as clearly, and performed poorly on simple memory tasks. Studies also show that people become better at remembering recently learned information after they have had a good night's sleep.

You don't need special equipment or workout clothes for tai chi. Wear loose, comfortable clothing that will not restrict your movements. Choose shoes with light support and thin, nonslip soles or just go barefoot.

Relieves stress. People who did tai chi for 18 weeks reduced levels of a stress hormone and reported lower levels of stress, a small German study found. During tai chi, you concentrate on breathing deeply and performing the movements. This has a calming effect that eases stress.

It may also help preserve your memory. Research suggests chronic life stress may lead to a decrease in the volume of the hippocampus, an area of your brain essential for learning and memory.

High levels of stress hormones have also been linked to poor memory, focus, and problem-solving skills. That barrage of stress hormones may shrink brain cells and disrupt connections between them. Tai chi not only helps prevent this, it may improve your energy and general mood.

Improves your memory. You can see how using tai chi to improve your sleep and stress levels may lead to better memory. But a pilot study suggests you can stave off memory loss more directly.

Researchers found that older adults who did tai chi scored just as well on memory tests as seniors who did aerobic exercise — and both groups scored better than exercise avoiders. In spite of its slow, gentle movements, tai chi qualifies as aerobic exercise. Researchers suspect you may get some of the same memory benefits from tai chi as you would from aerobic exercise, including these.

- More brain activity. Brain scans suggest aerobic exercise improves your brain activity and helps add brand new brain cells to your hippocampus. Not only are new brain cells good for thinking and memory, authorities say exercise may generate more new brain cells than anything else you can do.

- Less age-related memory loss. Aerobic exercise may delay the memory decline naturally caused by aging.

In addition to these benefits, some experts think the enjoyable mental effort of tai chi may deliver extra protection against dementia. But that's not all.

Research suggests tai chi may make your brain stronger and help stimulate your thinking ability. A small study found that older adults who participated in tai chi for just 10 weeks improved their "executive function," the vital mental ability involved in planning, organizing, paying attention to details, forming concepts, and thinking abstractly.

Defends against heart attacks and strokes. Studies suggest tai chi can help lower your blood pressure because it helps your blood vessels relax and dilate. Tai chi may also reduce your total cholesterol and raise your heart-protecting HDL cholesterol. Some experts think this happens because tai chi makes you more aerobically fit, which improves your cholesterol levels.

Improved blood pressure and cholesterol not only protect against heart attacks and strokes, they may also help prevent memory loss.

Several studies have linked high blood pressure to mental decline and memory problems. High blood pressure contributes to dementia because it restricts oxygen to the brain.

High cholesterol is just as bad. It can lead to plaque that clogs your arteries, meaning less oxygen-rich blood gets to your brain. If a clot forms and blocks the flow completely, you can suffer a heart attack or stroke.

When brain cells die from lack of oxygen or because of a clot-induced stroke, you can develop vascular dementia, the second most common dementia after AD. Strokes may also make your brain

Good news for anyone with diabetes or arthritis. You can find tai chi programs designed specifically to help you.

• Call 800-283-7800 or visit *www.arthritis.org* to find out if the Arthritis Foundation's tai chi program is available near you.

• Visit *www.amazon.com* for DVDs or books that can help you learn Dr. Paul Lam's tai chi program for diabetes. Ask your doctor if a "tai chi for diabetes" class is available locally.

produce beta-amyloid protein, a key component of the brain plaques found in people who have AD.

Fights diabetes. People who develop diabetes in mid-life may be more likely to have AD later in life. But tai chi may help lower blood sugar — and that might help you avoid both diabetes and dementia.

Find the best tai chi class for you

You can find tai chi lessons in books, DVDs, and even on the Internet but finding a class is still your best bet. Learning tai chi from a video or book means you can never be sure you are doing the movements correctly. Besides, learning tai chi with other people will be more fun.

Ask your doctor whether you can safely do tai chi. If she says yes, ask where to find a class suitable for you. If your doctor can't help, check your local senior center, nearby hospitals, or the YMCA. Also, get recommendations from your friends and family or visit *www.taichinetwork.org* to find schools and teachers near you.

Keep in mind that some tai chi classes may be more strenuous and complex than others. Before you commit to a class or instructor, check the cost of the classes and ask if you can watch one session to see if it has what you need.

Know when tai chi is unsafe

You may need to avoid certain forms, do a modified version of tai chi, or avoid tai chi completely if you have any of the following health issues — hernia, joint problems, back pain, sprains, fractures, or severe osteoporosis. Talk to your doctor to learn more.

Technology

Wii system • computer games
• handheld game units • smart phones

Stimulate your brain and get some exercise — all from the comfort of your living room. Today's technology can help you stay young and vibrant while you have fun. It's all about games for your mind and your body, along with new gadgets that let you play these games.

Playing games that challenge your brain can help you stay mentally young. The best choices are games that are new to you, giving you a workout in a critical area like visual-spatial skills, motor function, decision-making, language, or memory.

Research on people with dementia found certain computer games helped them keep their brains active and learn new skills. Experts say the mental stimulation needed to play games can give your brain just the workout it needs to stay in shape — whether or not you suffer from dementia. Improving how your brain works may help delay your brain's aging and improve your quality of life. The idea is that you build up a cognitive reserve, or savings account for your brain.

Certain games and gadgets, like Nintendo's Wii game system, let you get both mental and physical activity at once. Read on for more about four gadgets that let you play your way to brain health.

4 gadgets that keep you sharp

Wii game system. The Nintendo Wii game is a new kind of system. Unlike traditional video games, which involve mastering a complicated handheld controller, the Wii system uses a simple "wand" — a motion-sensing remote control — with just "A" and "B" buttons. Depending on the game, the controller transforms in your hand into a tennis racket, a baseball bat, a golf club, a bowling ball — the possibilities are almost endless. Some games also require an attached "nunchuck," a controller to hold in your other hand.

Wii is also different because many games on the system let you get physical. To play tennis, for example, you'll stand up, swing your "racket," and hit a virtual ball across a net on the screen.

Getting off the couch and into the game helps you stay mentally and physically young. Research shows being physically active has benefits for your brain, helping to slow its aging and decline while possibly boosting memory. One study showed getting a bit of physical activity can increase blood flow to your brain and help your thought processes. Older women in this study who were active, maybe taking a daily walk, showed better brain function than the inactive women.

Double your fun with a second Wii controller. The Wii game system comes with a single handheld controller and an attached controller for your other hand called a nunchuck. You need these to make the games work.

But if you want to play games like tennis or golf with a friend, it's worth buying a second set — controller and nunchuck. You can probably buy both for around $50. If your whole family will want to play at once, buy a few more sets.

Wii games are becoming quite popular at senior centers and senior housing complexes, where people seem to relish the opportunity to socialize and have fun together. You may even find a Wii bowling tournament at your local center, as some health care companies are donating systems for senior use. Playing in a group setting also helps you stay in touch with others and keeps your mind active.

One reason for Wii's popularity may be that games like boxing and tennis let you do activities you enjoyed when you were younger without the same risks of injury. You can even play the games while sitting down, using a flick of the wrist to fool the controller into thinking you're making larger motions. That means you can join in the fun — even if you have mobility problems.

Certain Wii games are not active but are designed specifically to give your brain a workout, like Big Brain Academy: Wii Degree.

Computer games. You can buy software packages that let you play games on your computer. But you may get tired of playing the same game repeatedly, and buying new ones can get expensive.

Many websites let you play games online for free. Some offer classic arcade games from the 1970s and 1980s — think favorites like Centipede or Missile Command. You can also find board games like chess and checkers, play card games including poker or bridge, work jigsaw puzzles or crossword puzzles, play trivia games, or try your hand at a war game. You can even play online against other people on their own computers, so you could, for example, play chess against your grandson in another state.

You'll find plenty of free game websites, but you may have to register or watch a brief advertisement before you play. Check out the games available on these websites.

- *www.addictinggames.com*

- *www.eons.com*

- *www.atari.com*

- *www.xgenstudios.com*

- *www.freewebarcade.com*

Handheld game systems. There's no need to invest in a computer to play computer games. Nifty little handheld systems let you join the fun and give your brain a workout. You can find inexpensive systems for less than $20 that let you play one or a few games, like sudoku or solitaire, at Wal-Mart, Target, or your local drugstore.

But if you want to invest in a handheld system that will let you play lots of well-written software and can connect with others on their handheld systems, consider a Nintendo DS. The new Nintendo DSi XL has a much larger screen than the original version. It costs about $190, including some game software. Expect to pay around $20 or more for each Nintendo DS game. Several target memory and brain skills.

Many games are available for more than one type of system, but they'll only work on the system they're designed for. If you want to buy Big Brain Academy for Wii, for example, be sure you don't accidentally pick up Big Brain Academy for Nintendo DS.

The same game sells at different prices depending on the system it's designed for. Consider that before you pick a game system.

- Brain Challenge

- Brain Age

- Puzzler World

Smart phones. When you carry an iPhone, Droid, or BlackBerry, you can do much more than just make phone calls. These smart phones transform into gaming machines when you load them with games or puzzles, sometimes called apps or "applications."

Hundreds of apps are available for you to download onto your smart phone, including some for free. Others typically cost less than $10. You'll find chess, poker, sudoku, billiards, and Monopoly, along with games intended to build your brain, like the math game Brain Twizzler. You can even test drive some apps before you buy them.

Check these sources for games and apps that will work on your phone.

- iPhone — Use the "Apple Store" link on your phone, or click on iTunes at *www.apple.com*.

- BlackBerry — Navigate to *www.appworld.com*.

- Droid — Use the "Android Market" link on your phone.

But a major drawback to playing games on a smart phone is the tiny screen, which seems created for younger eyes. Test the phone before you buy.

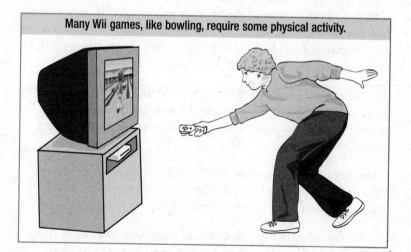
Many Wii games, like bowling, require some physical activity.

Skip the upgrade and save money

As new models of gadgets and game systems become available, you can find great deals on the old models.

For example, Nintendo's Wii system cost about $250 when it first came out. But now that some new games require the Wii balance board to play, you can pick up the basic system for less than $200. That's all you need to play classic games like boxing, bowling, or golf.

Same thing goes for other game systems, like the popular handheld Nintendo DS. You may even find a perfectly good used game system at some of the same stores that sell new ones. Try your local EB Games store or online retailers like *www.tigerdirect.com*.

Get the facts about cell phone risks

Could your mobile phone cause a tumor in your head?

Some research seems to show that people who use cell phones have a higher risk of tumors of the brain or salivary glands, especially on the side of your head where you hold your phone. Wireless phones emit nonionizing radiation, which is not known to damage cells or cause cancer. That's what the fuss is about.

Yet, other research shows no danger. Even more confusing, a recent international 10-year study, called the Interphone study, aiming to answer the question once and for all left its researchers debating what the results mean.

More research is being done, but it could be years before the experts know for sure how cell phones affect your brain. Until then, take these steps to lower the danger.

- Use a headset so you can hold the phone away from your head. Whether a wired headset or a Bluetooth wireless device, you're exposed to less radiation this way.

- Consider an air tube headset, which transmits sound waves to your ear through a plastic tube rather than through wires.

- Use the speakerphone option whenever possible to put some distance between the phone and your head.

- Shop for a phone with a low specific absorption rate (SAR). SAR is a measure of the level of radiation absorbed per kilogram of body weight.

- Keep calls short to limit your exposure time.

- Make calls when your phone's signal is strong. When it's poor, your phone compensates by raising the radiation level.

- Send a text message instead of calling when possible.

Thiamin

legumes • pork • enriched rice
• fortified cereals • nuts

Thiamin, also known as vitamin B1, may not be as famous as vitamin C or vitamin D, but you would be powerless without it. Just as electricity helps power the lights and appliances in your home, thiamin helps power your body.

Consider these examples of how thiamin keeps you going.

- helps your body turn fats and carbohydrates into energy

- works with other compounds to break down glucose, or blood sugar, a key fuel for your body

- assists in the Krebs cycle, a process that helps meet 90 percent of your energy needs

- helps your brain use blood sugar for fuel

- plays vital roles in your nerves and muscles, including your heart, and helps produce red blood cells

Be aware that thiamin is a water-soluble vitamin. That means your body does not store it to have on hand in case you run out — and you can run out of this vitamin in as little as 14 days.

Although thiamin deficiency is rare in the United States, certain groups still face a high risk. For example, older adults can become deficient because a medication keeps them from absorbing thiamin or because their diets are low in this vitamin. You may also be at risk if you:

- have had long-term dialysis or intravenous feeding.

- have diabetes.

- abuse alcohol.

- take diuretics.

- get most of your calories from carbohydrates, especially sugar or alcohol.

Mild symptoms of a thiamin deficiency include irritability, tiredness, and sleep disturbances. If a mild thiamin deficiency becomes severe, it is called beriberi. If you experience weight loss, fatigue, weakness, and loss of appetite, you may have beriberi. When beriberi isn't treated, your symptoms get worse and soon include nausea, depression, numbness, or paralysis.

To prevent this, you should aim for 1.2 milligrams (mg) of thiamin a day if you are a man and 1.1 mg a day if you are a woman. Eating thiamin-rich foods, like fortified breakfast cereal, oatmeal, pork, peas, and enriched white rice, can help.

Most people get enough thiamin from foods, so supplements are not usually necessary for healthy people eating a varied diet. However, if you suspect you need supplements, talk to your doctor first. Authorities have not set an upper limit on what you can safely take. Although thiamin is not thought to be toxic, very high doses can cause stomach upset.

Also, be aware that thiamin comes in several forms. Thiamin hydrochloride, thiamin nitrate, and thiamin mononitrate are water soluble,

3/4 cup Total whole-grain breakfast cereal	1.5 mg*
3 oz. pork chops	1 mg
1 cup trail mix with chocolate chips, salted nuts, and seeds	0.6 mg
3 oz. roasted, cured ham	0.57 mg
1 enriched plain or sesame 4-inch bagel	0.53 mg
1 cup Kellogg's Special K cereal	0.52 mg
1 cup boiled black-eyed peas without salt	0.45 mg
1 cup parboiled, enriched long-grain white rice	0.37 mg
1 cup roasted chestnuts	0.34 mg

* milligrams

but benfotiamine is a fat-soluble version your body can store. Ask your doctor about the differences between these versions.

2 ways thiamin keeps you sharp

Fights diabetic atherosclerosis. You are more likely to be deficient in thiamin if you have diabetes than if you have normal blood sugar, one study recently found. Even when people with diabetes get enough thiamin from food, they are likely to be deficient because their bodies get rid of it through the urine at an astonishing rate.

This shortage means blood vessel cells do not have enough thiamin. If you have diabetes, this may interfere with your blood vessels' ability to dilate when they should.

That may raise your risk of atherosclerosis, the buildup of fatty deposits called plaques on your artery walls. When arteries are narrowed, less oxygen-rich blood can circulate through them. If the plaques burst, they can cause a blood clot. If a clot forms and blocks off blood flow completely, you may suffer a heart attack or stroke.

This is bad news for your brain in two ways. When brain cells die due to a lack of oxygen or because of a clot-induced stroke, you can develop vascular dementia, the second most common dementia after Alzheimer's

> Medications like digoxin (Lanoxin), phenytoin (Dilantin), and furosemide (Lasix) or other diuretics may reduce your thiamin levels. In fact, Digoxin may even affect your heart's ability to use thiamin. If you take one of these medications, ask your doctor if you need a thiamin supplement.

disease (AD.) In addition, strokes can trigger your brain to produce more beta-amyloid plaques, which are key components of AD.

A small study suggests added thiamin may help restore your blood vessels' ability to dilate properly. That may help prevent atherosclerosis or slow its progress — and may fend off its brain-threatening results, too. If you have diabetes, talk to your doctor about whether you need thiamin supplements.

Resists dementia. You might not expect thiamin deficiency to have a link to Alzheimer's, but studies have noted at least two possible connections.

- More plaques. Plaques made of beta-amyloid protein appear in the brain when a person has AD. Doctors don't know if these plaques cause AD or are caused by it, but the plaques block brain cells from connecting with one another. When they cannot communicate, they die and brain tissue shrinks. One animal study found that thiamin deficiency increased the amount of brain space plagued by plaques and raised the amount of beta-amyloid protein in the brain.

- More brain malfunctions. Remember the energy crisis of the 70s? The brain experiences something similar as dementia develops. Your brain uses glucose as fuel. But as dementia progresses, the brain's ability to make use of glucose dwindles. Experts call this "reduced glucose metabolism," and it's considered a symptom of Alzheimer's. Processes that depend on thiamin play a key role in glucose metabolism. But in people with Alzheimer's, thiamin processes are impaired. This is bad news because a reduction in these processes has also been linked with free radical damage, a long-suspected cause of AD.

Over the years, several studies have tested thiamin supplements against AD, but most have met with little or no success. Scientists say they need more information to accurately determine whether or not thiamin works. Because thiamin comes in several different forms, some experts have also wondered whether the right kind of thiamin was used.

A recent animal study tried the fat-soluble version of thiamin, benfotiamine. Their results suggest benfotiamine can improve spatial memory and reduce beta-amyloid plaques. More research is needed to determine whether benfotiamine can produce the same results in people, so stay tuned.

Find the best supplement

If you have a thiamin deficiency, you may also be deficient in other B vitamins. That's because most B vitamins come from the same food groups. If your doctor approves a thiamin supplement, ask if you need a multivitamin or B complex vitamin that includes all eight B vitamins — thiamin, riboflavin, niacin, pantothenic acid, vitamin B6, vitamin B12, biotin, and folate.

Because recent consumer testing revealed that some B vitamin supplements don't contain the amounts promised on their labels, ask your doctor which supplement she recommends.

Simple secrets prevent deficiency

Getting more thiamin may be easier than you think. Try these tips to help you boost your thiamin intake.

- Microwave foods or choose sources of thiamin that need no cooking, such as bagels, nuts, and fortified, ready-to-eat breakfast cereals. Heating food destroys thiamin, but microwaving food does less damage.

- Go easy on tea and coffee. Drinking lots of tea and coffee can make your body absorb less thiamin — even decaf.

- Smoking makes your body absorb and use less thiamin. That's another great reason to quit.

Little-known herbal interaction

What you take for incontinence could put you at risk for a thiamin deficiency. Here's why. Some herbal supplement formulas for incontinence include the herb horsetail. Check the ingredient list on the bottle to see if yours is one of them.

Horsetail contains an enzyme that can destroy thiamin. Some horsetail products contain this enzyme while others do not. Before you take horsetail and thiamin together, ask your doctor or pharmacist which preparations of horsetail to use.

Vitamin B12

dairy • fish • shellfish • meat
• fortified breakfast cereals

Forgetful lately? You could have a simple vitamin deficiency. B12
works closely with folate, helping its fellow B-vitamin build
healthy red blood cells, and
preserves the sheaths
surrounding nerve fibers.

Up to 90 percent of people
deficient in B12 develop
neurologic symptoms such as
weakness, numbness, tingling,
or paralysis, but other signs can
be more subtle. Too little B12
may contribute to forgetfulness,
depression, dementia, brain
shrinkage, and insufficient
blood flow to the brain — the
main cause of strokes.

Could you soon be at risk for
memory loss? Science suggests
that many people, especially

3 oz. steamed blue crab	6.21 mcg*
1 cup Total Raisin Bran	6.0 mcg
3 oz. cooked rainbow trout	4.22 mcg
3 oz. canned salmon with bones	3.74 mcg
3 oz. cooked ground beef patty	2.24 mcg
1 cup low-fat cottage cheese	1.42 mcg
8 oz. plain, fat-free yogurt	1.38 mcg
1 cup skim milk	1.23 mcg

* micrograms

seniors, don't have enough B12 in their system. As many as one in
five elderly adults are deficient. Certain people need this B-vitamin
more than others. See if you're in one of these high-risk categories.

- Strict vegetarians, known as vegans, face a serious risk for
  vitamin B12 deficiency. They must take supplements since
  only animal foods naturally contain this nutrient.

- Some elderly adults have trouble absorbing B12 from food, generally thanks to atrophic gastritis. This condition causes chronic inflammation of the stomach lining, limiting the amount of acid your stomach produces. Without enough, your stomach cannot release the B12 trapped in food, and your body can't absorb it.

- People with pernicious anemia don't make enough stomach acid, either. In this illness, your immune system attacks and destroys the acid-secreting cells that line your stomach. About one in 50 people over age 60 suffer from this condition, as do one in five of their relatives.

- Medications that reduce stomach acid, such as omeprazole (Prilosec) and ranitidine (Zantac), can make it hard to get enough B12 from food, for the same reason.

- Other drugs can block your body from absorbing this vitamin, too, including colchicine for gout, oral diabetes drugs such as metformin and phenformin, and slow-release potassium supplements.

- People taking folic acid supplements risk developing severe B12 deficiency. Folate can disguise the symptoms of a B12 shortage. Without the normal warning signs, you may not realize you're deficient until you have developed permanent nerve damage. For this reason, experts warn against taking high doses of folic acid without a doctor's supervision.

People over age 50 need 2.4 micrograms (mcg) of B12 daily to stave off obvious deficiency. However, some experts argue that's a minimum and not enough for good health. In one study, women who got between 3 and 6 mcg of vitamin B12 daily still showed signs of deficiency. Those who got more than 6 mcg daily did not.

Fortunately, you can do something about it quickly. Your body absorbs the B12 in some foods better than in others. Scientists call this "bioavailability." New evidence shows milk boasts the most bioavailable B12, although heating it does destroy some of the vitamin. Cottage cheese, hard cheese, and blue cheese also contain B12.

Raw meat packs a lot, too, but meat loses around one-third of its B12 when you cook it. Plus, some people have trouble absorbing this vitamin from meat. The B12 in fish is more bioavailable. Even when cooked, salmon, trout, tuna, and sardines are top-notch sources. So are oysters, mussels, and clams. Breakfast cereals fortified with B12 can help close the nutritional gap.

4 ways vitamin B12 keeps you sharp

Slows memory loss. Low levels of this vitamin led to faster mental decline over 10 years for a group of seniors age 65 and older. That's a real problem, because B12 shortages are especially common in older adults, and they become more common with age.

Doubling your blood levels of this vitamin could slow mental decline by one-third. In another study, people with higher levels of vitamins B12 and B6 had more grey matter in the parts of the brain associated with memory, attention, and organization.

Based on research, you would need 250 micrograms (mcg) of this nutrient daily for 16 weeks to double your B12 levels. That's roughly 100 times the Recommended Dietary

Even healthy people can only absorb so much B12 at a time, generally no more than 2 micrograms (mcg) per meal. Eat foods rich in this vitamin throughout the day, not just at one meal, to reach your daily goals. Start the morning with a bowl of fortified cereal, enjoy grilled salmon for lunch, and have a glass of low-fat milk before bed.

Allowance. Start by building more B12 into your diet naturally, then talk to your doctor about whether you need supplements.

Derails dementia. This brain-building vitamin slashes blood levels of homocysteine, an amino acid linked to Alzheimer's, heart disease, and brain shrinkage.

- A shortage of B vitamins, including B12, B6, and folate, sends homocysteine levels climbing and speeds up the development of Alzheimer's-like plaques in mice.

- Science also links high homocysteine levels with faster brain shrinkage. People with confirmed cases of Alzheimer's disease (AD) tend to have brain shrinkage, and as the shrinking worsens so does AD.

You don't need a severe B12 shortage to face a danger, either. Even slightly low levels of this precious nutrient can affect your brain. A study of people 61 to 87 years old linked low B12 levels to brain shrinkage over five years. No one in this study qualified as B12-deficient. Their blood levels were low but still in the normal range, suggesting even a slight shortage may put you at risk for mental decline.

> Protect your brain by bumping your B12 levels into the normal range naturally. Foods like a turkey sandwich may help the elderly avoid mental decline, with its balance of both B12 and folate. Turkey and cheese boast a fine share of B12, while lettuce and fortified bread deliver a healthy dose of folate.

Experts think low B12 may lead to inflammation in your brain or damage to the delicate sheaths surrounding brain and nerve cells. The good news — boosting your B12 levels from low-normal may prevent further brain shrinkage.

Stops stroke. People with heart disease who took a combination of B12, B6, and folic acid for five years were less likely to suffer a disabling stroke. Once again, the benefit was probably due to a drop in homocysteine.

It took about three years for the protection to kick in, but the wait could be worth it for some people. The impact on stroke risk was biggest for people who:

- were under 70 years old.

- started out with high cholesterol or homocysteine levels.

- were not taking antiplatelet or cholesterol-lowering drugs.

While B-vitamin therapy may help prevent first-time strokes, it may not ward off future ones.

Lifts depression. Getting more vitamins B12 and B6 may cut your risk of depression. Depression by itself is bad enough, but it boosts your risk for Alzheimer's disease, too. People with a history of depression are two to four times more likely to develop AD later in life.

Vitamin B12 deficiency could be a major culprit. Women with a B12 deficiency were twice as likely to suffer from severe depression in one study, and as many as 30 percent of people hospitalized for depression are low in B12. Your body needs B12 to make the compound SAMe, and it uses SAMe to make chemical messengers in your brain. Having too few messengers may lead to depression.

For every 10 mcg more of B12 people received daily, their odds of becoming depressed dropped 2 percent. While this vitamin won't necessarily cure the illness, experts do suggest asking your doctor to test your B12 levels if you struggle with depression.

Best ways to beat a B12 shortage

Some people need supplements to get enough vitamin B12, either because their current levels are so low or because they have trouble absorbing it from food.

Ask your doctor to test your B12 levels. The results will help determine if you need supplements and what kind. Some people do fine taking B12 by mouth while others will need injections.

- Injections can quickly treat a deficiency. Since they bypass your stomach, they get around any problems you may have absorbing this vitamin.

- High dosages of B12 taken by mouth may work, too. Your doctor will decide on the dosage.

Experts say people over age 50 may need fortified cereals and supplements to get enough B12 every day. Keep in mind, some B12 supplements also contain folic acid, and too much of it can worsen the symptoms of B12 deficiency. Consider a B12-only supplement if necessary.

Balance your B vitamins for brain health

The B vitamins B12 and folate both help keep your mind keen, but only if you get a healthy balance of them. Too much folate and too little B12 could dull your brain and speed up mental decline.

Excess folate can aggravate the symptoms of B12 deficiency in seniors. People with high folate but normal B12 levels are less likely to develop cognitive impairment — problems with memory, judgment, and perception — or anemia, two trademarks of a B12 shortage. High folate and low B12, however, spells trouble. People with this combination were five times more likely to suffer from cognitive impairment and anemia.

This imbalance may speed up mental decline, too. Some research links high folate plus low B12 to a faster rate of mental decline in older adults.

About one in five seniors have high blood levels of folate, largely thanks to supplements containing folic acid. Check labels. Avoid getting more than 400 micrograms of folic acid a day from supplements, including multivitamins.

Vitamin B6

fish • fortified cereals • banana • spinach • greens • bell peppers • cabbage • celery

Vitamin B6 doesn't get much respect. It's a workhorse vitamin, like the busy innkeeper with a hand in every job around the place, yet nobody notices. In fact, vitamin B6 has an effect on more than 60 proteins in your body, including some important for your heart, nervous system, and blood cell production.

Your body needs vitamin B6, or pyridoxine, for various enzymes to function and for the production of some phospholipids, major building blocks of cell membranes, and amino acids. Vitamin B6 also helps your body make

4 oz. baked yellowfin tuna	1.18 mg*
1 cup Wheaties	1 mg
1 banana	0.68 mg
4 oz. baked cod	0.52 mg
1 cup cooked spinach	0.44 mg
1 cup cooked turnip greens	0.26 mg
1 cup red bell peppers	0.23 mg
1 cup cooked cabbage	0.17 mg
1 cup celery	0.10 mg

* milligrams

neurotransmitters — messenger chemicals that help your nervous system work — like serotonin, dopamine, norepinephrine, and gamma-amino butyric acid (GABA).

Vitamin B6 is especially important because of its response to homocysteine, a real bad guy in the world of health. This amino acid damages blood cells and increases your risk of dangerous clots. Because of this, high levels of homocysteine are linked to both dementia and heart disease. Homocysteine forms when your body breaks down certain compounds. But vitamin B6 acts as a bouncer, removing excess homocysteine from your body.

You may see vitamin B6 referred to by its various forms:

- pyridoxine
- pyridoxal
- pyridoxamine
- pyridoxine phosphate
- pyridoxal phosphate
- pyridoxamine phosphate

Deficiency of vitamin B6 is rare, occurring mostly in alcoholics. The classic signs of deficiency show up first on your skin, like seborrheic dermatitis or eczema. Other problems include nervous system disorders like memory problems, irritability, and depression; higher levels of homocysteine; and a raised risk of kidney stones. You may also notice inflammation of your tongue and sores in and around your mouth.

The daily recommended intake for vitamin B6 is 1.3 milligrams (mg) for adults younger than age 50, 1.5 mg for women over age 50, and 1.7 mg for men over age 50.

It's difficult to get too much vitamin B6 from food. Like other water-soluble vitamins, extra vitamin B6 is flushed out of your body. An excess from supplements, however, can lead to nerve damage. Too much may cause sensory neuropathy, characterized by pain and numbness in your extremities and difficulty walking. That usually happens only at high doses of more than 1,000 mg a day for several months.

5 ways vitamin B6 keeps you sharp

Staves off the blues. Experts think low levels of vitamin B6, vitamin B12, and folic acid may lead to depression. Your brain needs a constant supply of the right vitamins to function and keep your mood stable. You need vitamin B6 to make neurotransmitters that help regulate mood, but studies on B vitamins have been conflicting.

Research on people age 65 and older in Chicago found those who get more vitamin B6 and vitamin B12 have a lower risk of depression. This study boosts the theory that taking supplements of vitamin B6 — alone or with other B vitamins — may help with mood.

Saves your sight. Vitamin B6 also plays a role in preventing age-related macular degeneration (AMD). This major cause of blindness among seniors develops slowly, damaging your eye's macula, which is responsible for providing color and detail to your central vision.

Women who took 50 milligrams (mg) of vitamin B6, along with vitamin B12 and folic acid, daily for seven years were up to 40 percent less likely to develop AMD. Experts think the vitamin trio breaks down and eliminates homocysteine from your body. This naturally occurring amino acid damages the lining of your blood vessels and raises your risk of blood clots. Also, the three B vitamins are antioxidants and protect the fragile photoreceptors in your eyes.

Researchers have also noticed a link between eye disease and problems with thinking and memory. One study of seniors found those with the poorest scores on a standardized test of mental skills were twice as likely to have early AMD. Experts don't fully understand the link. If you have either condition — dementia or AMD — get screened for the other.

Helps your heart. People with more of the active form of vitamin B6, called pyridoxal-5-phosphate (PLP), in their blood are at a lower risk of diabetes, obesity, and metabolic syndrome, which includes high blood sugar, abdominal fat, high blood pressure, and high cholesterol. That's because more PLP means you probably have less C-reactive protein in your blood, meaning less inflammation.

The effect of vitamin B6 on homocysteine levels also makes it a big player in preventing heart disease and stroke. A five-year study of people who already had heart disease found the combination of vitamin B6, vitamin B12, and folic acid seemed to lower both their homocysteine levels and their risk of stroke. Just 50 mg of vitamin B6 in the combo lowered chances of a stroke by about 25 percent.

Other studies have had similar positive results with B vitamins lowering the risk of stroke, heart disease, and heart failure, although some research shows no heart protection.

If you and your doctor decide you need supplements of vitamin B6 and other B vitamins, you can save money and hassle by taking the big players all in a single pill.

Brands including Holista, Sundown Naturals, and Mason Natural make single pills that contain vitamin B6, vitamin B12, and folic acid — a common combination. You could save more than 25 percent by purchasing a combination supplement.

Don't take more than 100 milligrams of vitamin B6 daily without talking to your doctor.

Puts the brakes on Parkinson's. Loss of the neurotransmitter dopamine is a key feature of Parkinson's disease. Dopamine affects movement, coordination, and information processing in your brain. That's why people suffering from Parkinson's may have tremors, slow movement, poor balance, and trouble walking, along with difficulty thinking, talking, and remembering.

There's only a little research to show a link, but getting too little vitamin B6 in your diet may put you at higher risk of Parkinson's. Again, the connection is homocysteine levels. Experts suspect too much homocysteine may kill off cells that make dopamine, bringing on Parkinson's.

Heads off Alzheimer's. The homocysteine link also may mean getting enough vitamin B6 — along with its fabulous friends vitamin B12 and folic acid — could help stave off Alzheimer's disease. Research on mice shows a connection between the vitamins, a buildup of homocysteine, and Alzheimer-like symptoms. Researchers are continuing to look into the connection.

Beware vitamin-leaching drugs	
Some common prescription drugs can deplete vitamin B6 from your body.	
Drug	**What it's for**
furosemide (Lasix)	loop diuretic or water pill
hydralazine (Apresoline)	high blood pressure
penicillamine (Cuprimine)	rheumatoid arthritis
gentamicin	bacterial infections
theophylline (Bronkodyl)	bronchitis, emphysema, asthma
carbamazepine (Carbatrol)	anti-epileptic
phenobarbital (Luminal)	barbiturate sedative
oral estrogen	hormone-replacement therapy

Keep a lid on vitamins

Cooking and processing, including canning and freezing, can take out a lot of vitamin B6 from food.

Keep this rule in mind — the more acidic the food, the more vitamin B6 is lost when you cook it. Even freezing causes a loss of one-third to one-half of a food's vitamin B6.

Make up for this loss by eating lots of foods rich in vitamin B6. Although most foods high in this important vitamin need to be cooked, there are a few exceptions, like bell peppers and celery. Eat them raw for more B6.

Lack of vitamin B6 can lead to lowered immunity, especially in seniors. The problem is caused when your body doesn't produce enough of the immune system protein interleukin-2 and lymphocytes, white blood cells that aid immunity.

One study found that seniors need more vitamin B6 than the Recommended Dietary Allowance (RDA) to restore a strong immune system after a deficiency. Men may need 2.9 milligrams (mg) a day, while women need 1.9 mg a day. Talk to your doctor before you take a high dose.

Vitamin C

citrus fruits • strawberries • papaya • tomatoes
• potatoes • broccoli • bell peppers • brussels sprouts
• leafy green vegetables • fortified breakfast cereals

Time was running out for French explorer Jacques Cartier and his crew. The year was 1536. They were marooned in the Canadian wilderness for the winter, and they were dying from a severe vitamin C deficiency called scurvy. Amazingly, friendly Canadian Indians arrived and suggested making a tea from the leaves and bark of a nearby tree. Every man who drank the tea recovered because the tea was rich in vitamin C.

Vitamin C is just as important to your health as it was to Cartier's men. Here are just a few reasons why.

- Your body uses vitamin C to make collagen, important for wound healing and a crucial building block for blood vessels, skin, cartilage, tendons, and ligaments. Collagen also helps repair and maintain your teeth and bones.

- Vitamin C helps produce several compounds vital to normal brain function. In fact, high amounts of vitamin C can be found in your brain.

- Vitamin C is an antioxidant that can fend off damage from free radical molecules. Free radical damage plays a role in heart disease, Alzheimer's, and other health problems.

- You need vitamin C to make L-carnitine, a compound that helps convert fat into energy.

- Vitamin C is a major player in your immune system.

You can see why experts say you need 75 milligrams (mg) of vitamin C every day if you are a woman or 90 mg if you are a man. Although many Americans get enough vitamin C, up to 14 percent do not. You may be more likely to come up short if you:

- eat a limited variety of foods.

- smoke or are exposed to secondhand smoke.

- have a condition that prevents you from absorbing nutrients well.

Signs you need more vitamin C include fatigue, gum inflammation, and feeling unwell. Over time, you may also develop joint pain, skin problems, easy bruising or bleeding, dry and splitting hair, depression, bleeding gums, tooth loss or loose teeth, and hair loss.

Eat 2 1/2 cups of fruits and veggies a day, and you can get up to 200 mg of vitamin C. But keep in mind that light, air, lengthy storage, and heat can cause foods to lose vitamin C. To get the most vitamin C from your diet, eat foods raw, microwaved, or lightly steamed.

4 ways vitamin C keeps you sharp

Curbs high blood pressure. Experts say higher blood pressure has been linked with vitamin C deficiency. Vitamin C helps keep your blood vessels flexible, which may help lower blood pressure. If you don't get enough vitamin C and your blood pressure rises, your brain may pay the price.

Recent studies suggest high blood pressure may damage the tiny blood vessels that nourish your brain's white matter, the network of nerve fibers that helps brain cells communicate. This leads to white matter lesions, a type of scarring linked to Alzheimer's disease (AD) and other forms of dementia. The higher your blood pressure and the longer it goes uncontrolled, the more white matter damage occurs.

1 papaya	187 mg*
1 cup freshly squeezed orange juice	124 mg
1 cup cranberry juice cocktail	107 mg
1 cup boiled broccoli	101.2 mg
1 cup strawberries	97.6 mg
1/2 cup sweet red peppers	95.1 mg
1 cup Kellogg's Product 19 cereal	61.2 mg

* milligrams

Slices stroke risk. Getting too little vitamin C has been linked with a higher risk of stroke. That is bad news because a stroke can also raise your risk of dementia.

During a stroke, blood vessels become blocked or burst, cutting off blood flow to part of your brain and killing brain cells. When brain cells die, your risk of vascular dementia rises. Strokes may also trigger processes linked to AD.

Guards against heart disease. People with lower blood levels of vitamin C face a higher risk of heart disease, heart attacks, and even peripheral artery disease (PAD). But vitamin C may help protect your heart by protecting your arteries. If your "bad" LDL cholesterol gets damaged by free radicals, it may gradually build up on the inner walls of the arteries that feed your heart and brain. Over time, this damaged LDL forms plaque, a thick, hard deposit that narrows your arteries and makes them less flexible. Doctors call this atherosclerosis. If a clot forms and blocks the flow completely, you can suffer a heart attack or stroke.

> Try this easy way to cut back on sodium. Read vitamin C supplement labels and choose calcium ascorbate or ascorbic acid instead of sodium ascorbate. Every 1,000 milligrams (mg) of sodium ascorbate adds 131 mg of sodium to your daily total.

Vitamin C may help prevent atherosclerosis by protecting LDL from becoming damaged in the first place. What's more, this vitamin may also prevent several other processes that lead to atherosclerosis. So getting enough vitamin C may help you avoid heart disease and heart attacks. This is important because people who have heart disease and high cholesterol have a significantly higher risk of dementia.

Fends off obesity. People who take in too little vitamin C may be more likely to become obese, preliminary evidence suggests. This is what studies say so far.

- The lower your blood levels of vitamin C, the heavier you are likely to be.

- People who took vitamin C supplements were able to lose more weight in six weeks than people who didn't take the supplements.

- Lower blood levels of vitamin C have been linked to a higher percentage of body fat in women and to bigger waists and a higher body mass index, which is used to estimate a healthy weight based on your height, in both genders.

Vitamin C is vital to your body's ability to make L-carnitine, a compound you need to burn fat. In fact, early studies suggest people who barely get enough vitamin C burn less fat during exercise. More research is needed to determine whether vitamin C truly affects your weight. But if vitamin C does help you control your weight, it may also help you avoid dementia.

If you are a woman carrying too many pounds, you are twice as likely to have dementia as a woman at a healthy weight. If you carry that weight mostly around your middle, you almost triple your odds of developing dementia. If you are overweight, you are also more likely to have higher C-reactive protein (CRP) levels. CRP is associated with thinking and memory problems, as well as dementia.

> The antioxidant powers of vitamin C do more than just protect your brain. When combined with other antioxidants, this vitamin may help protect your eyesight from the diseases of old age. Learn more about this in the *Age-related macular degeneration* chapter.

Get more bang for your vitamin C buck

Start with these tips to get the most benefits from your vitamin C supplement.

- Take vitamin C supplements in small doses two or three times a day with meals.

- Drink plenty of water and make sure a bathroom is available when taking vitamin C supplements. Vitamin C can act as a diuretic.

- Don't overdo it. People who take in 30 to 180 milligrams (mg) of vitamin C a day absorb 70 to 90 percent of that vitamin C. But people who take in 1,000 mg a day may only absorb 50 percent. If you have taken high doses of vitamin C for a long time and want to cut back, do so gradually or your blood levels of vitamin C may fall too low.

5 hidden dangers you should know about

Vitamin C supplements can have unexpected and sometimes dangerous effects on your body. Before you swallow a supplement, take precautions like these.

- High doses of this vitamin may interfere with lab tests. Make sure your doctor knows how much vitamin C you take.

- Talk to your doctor before taking a vitamin C supplement, especially if you take nonsteroidal anti-inflammatory drugs (NSAIDs) like aspirin or ibuprofen, aluminum-based antacids, acetaminophen, chemotherapy drugs, nitrate medications for heart disease, tetracycline, or blood thinners like warfarin.

- Protect yourself from a vitamin B12 deficiency. Taking too much vitamin C may prevent your body from absorbing vitamin B12.

> Make an extra effort to get enough vitamin C if you struggle with low iron levels. Vitamin C can help your body absorb more iron.

- If your doctor approves a vitamin C supplement, you can choose from tablets, capsules, chewable, liquids, and effervescent forms of the vitamin. Keep in mind frequent use of chewable vitamin C can cause tooth erosion.

- High amounts of vitamin C may cause side effects. If vitamin C supplements cause diarrhea, heartburn, gas, and other digestive symptoms, try a lower dose. If your doctor has recommended a high dose, read labels and switch to the sodium ascorbate or calcium ascorbate form of vitamin C. These "buffered" versions may be gentler to your stomach than ascorbic acid. The Institute of Medicine has set the tolerable upper intake level for vitamin C at 2,000 mg.

Vitamin D

fortified milk • fortified cereal • salmon
• tuna • mackerel • beef liver • cheese
• egg yolks • mushrooms • flaxseeds

"On the Sunny Side of the Street" is not just a popular song from the great American songbook. It's also a good place to get vitamin D.

That's because your skin produces vitamin D when it's exposed to sunlight. Nicknamed "the sunshine vitamin," vitamin D performs several functions in your body. Most notably, it helps you absorb calcium and build and strengthen bones. It also helps your muscles move, your nerves transmit messages, and your immune system fight off infection.

The childhood disease rickets, marked by soft bones, is caused by vitamin D deficiency. Adults who don't get enough vitamin D could develop osteomalacia — a painful condition involving soft, spongy bones — or osteoporosis.

But vitamin D may be even more essential. Recently, scientists have linked low vitamin D levels to several conditions, including heart disease, diabetes, certain cancers, chronic pain, arthritis, gum disease, and dementia.

In addition to sunlight, you can get vitamin D from certain foods. Fatty fish, like salmon, herring, mackerel, sardines, and tuna, are your best bets. Fortified foods, such as milk and cereal, also provide vitamin D. You can even get a small amount from egg yolks and cheese. But to get enough vitamin D, you may need to take supplements.

3 oz. salmon	794 IU*
3 oz. tuna, canned in oil	229 IU
3 oz. sardines, canned in oil	164 IU
1 cup fortified whole milk	124 IU
1 cup fortified fat-free or skim milk	115 IU
1 cup Total Raisin Bran	104 IU
1 cup cooked shiitake mushrooms	45 IU
1 large scrambled egg	29 IU

* international units

There are two types of vitamin D supplements — vitamin D2 (ergocalciferol) and vitamin D3 (cholecalciferol). Vitamin D3 is the form that's most useful for your body. When buying supplements, look for vitamin D3 on the label.

However you get your vitamin D, it must undergo a few changes to be activated in your body. The first change happens in your liver, where vitamin D is converted to 25-hydroxyvitamin D, or 25(OH)D. Your doctor may measure your blood levels of 25(OH)D to determine your vitamin D status. The other change takes place in your kidneys, resulting in the active form of vitamin D called 1,25-dihydroxyvitamin D, or 1,25(OH)2D.

How much vitamin D do you need? The recommended intake of vitamin D is 400 International Units (IU) for people over age 50 and 600 IU for people over age 70, but many experts say that's too low. Older people, people who live in northern climates, and people with dark skin may need more. Many health professionals say you should aim for at least 1,000 IU a day.

Chances are you're not getting enough of this important vitamin. But spending a little more time in the sun, eating foods rich in vitamin D, and supplementing your diet can make a big difference. Boost your vitamin D levels to give your brain — and overall health — a boost.

5 ways vitamin D keeps you sharp

Defeats dementia. Your golden years can be sunnier with vitamin D. Upping your levels of this key vitamin may help stave off mental decline and dementia, including Alzheimer's disease.

One six-year study of older people — age 65 and up — in Italy found that those with very low vitamin D levels were more likely to experience declines in thinking, learning, and memory than those with sufficient vitamin D levels.

Similar results were found in a study of 3,325 older people in the United States. Low vitamin D levels meant a higher risk for mental impairment, as measured by tests of memory, orientation in time and space, and attention. People who were severely deficient in vitamin D were more than four times more likely to be mentally impaired than those with normal levels.

A British study found that low blood levels of vitamin D may boost your risk for dementia. In a study of older people, those with the lowest levels of vitamin D were 2.3 times more likely to have mental impairment compared to those with the highest levels.

In another study, older people with high levels of vitamin D performed better on tests of "executive function" — the mental ability involved in planning, organizing, paying attention to details, forming concepts, and thinking abstractly. They were also less likely to have damage to small blood vessels in the brain or disease in the brain's white matter.

While no direct link has been established, receptors for vitamin D have been found in the areas of the brain involved in complex planning, processing, and the formation of new memories.

British researchers found that men with higher levels of vitamin D performed better on a test that measures attention and speed of processing information. The link was stronger in men over age 60.

Laboratory tests suggest that vitamin D protects neurons, supports brain function, and reduces inflammation. One lab study found that vitamin D3 may help prevent the buildup of beta-amyloid protein in the brain by stimulating macrophages, your immune system's garbage men, to absorb and remove it.

> Put away those pain pills. Vitamin D may be just what the doctor ordered. Studies show that people with chronic body aches and back pain usually have low levels of vitamin D. Luckily, those aches and pains often diminish or disappear once you start getting enough vitamin D.

Prevents Parkinson's. Parkinson's disease comes with several symptoms, including tremors, stooped posture, slow movement, poor balance, and a shuffling walk. You can add low vitamin D levels to the list. In fact, low vitamin D levels may play a role in the development of this condition.

Emory University researchers discovered that people with Parkinson's disease were more likely to have insufficient levels of vitamin D than healthy people or those with Alzheimer's disease. Because of mobility problems, people with Parkinson's might get less sun exposure, which could explain the difference. But low vitamin D levels may also contribute to Parkinson's, and boosting your intake may help.

A Finnish study with a 29-year follow-up period found that people with higher vitamin D levels were less likely to develop Parkinson's disease. People with the highest levels were 67 percent less likely to develop Parkinson's than those with the lowest.

How exactly vitamin D may help protect against Parkinson's remains unclear, but researchers point to its antioxidant activity, ability to regulate calcium levels, detoxification powers, and effect on the immune system as possibilities.

Destroys depression. Brighten your mood with bright sunshine. Getting more vitamin D may help you clear the dark clouds of depression.

A six-year study of people in Tuscany age 65 or older found that those with low vitamin D levels were more likely to become depressed. The link was stronger for women, but also applied to men. Another study of people with heart disease found that those with low vitamin D levels were more likely to be depressed.

Dutch researchers found that older people with depression had lower blood levels of vitamin D. Lower vitamin D levels also meant more severe depression.

But the link between vitamin D and depression has a certain chicken-or-egg aspect. Are you depressed because you have low vitamin D levels or do you have low vitamin D levels because you're depressed? If you're depressed, you may be less likely to leave your house, so you get less exposure to sunshine. You may also neglect to eat a healthy diet, depriving yourself of good food sources of vitamin D.

Getting more vitamin D may be an easy way to improve your mental health. Fish has long been recommended for its omega-3 fatty acids — but the vitamin D in fish could also help with depression.

Hampers heart disease. An unhealthy heart often means an unhealthy brain. Fortunately, your brain can take heart in vitamin D's protective powers.

An analysis of 28 studies found that people with high levels of vitamin D reduced their risk for heart disease by 33 percent. They also reduced their risk of developing diabetes by 55 percent and metabolic syndrome by 51 percent.

On the other hand, low levels of vitamin D spell trouble for your heart — and your life. In one study, people with the lowest vitamin D levels were twice as likely to die of any cause as those with higher levels. But the risk of heart-related death was even greater.

> Keep your balance by keeping your vitamin D levels up to par. A recent review of eight studies found that people age 65 and older who took 700 to 1,000 IU of vitamin D each day reduced their risk of falling by 19 to 26 percent.

Men with low vitamin D levels were more than twice as likely to have a heart attack as those with normal levels, according to another study. Low vitamin D has also been linked to high blood pressure. One study even determined that men with vitamin D deficiency were more than five times more likely to develop high blood pressure as those with sufficient levels.

Vitamin D may also help counteract the inflammation associated with congestive heart failure.

Dampens diabetes. Diabetes means more than high blood sugar. It also means a higher risk for heart problems, obesity, and dementia. Vitamin D — think D for diabetes — may help.

Studies suggest that low vitamin D levels are common in people with diabetes — and possibly a risk factor for developing the condition. Low vitamin D levels have also been linked to poor blood sugar control and insulin resistance.

Other studies show that supplemental vitamin D can help reduce the risk of diabetes and insulin resistance.

Succeed with supplements and sunshine

Up to half of all adults have less than optimum levels of vitamin D. But people are starting to catch on. In a recent survey by Consumer Lab, vitamin D ranked as the fifth most-popular supplement.

Luckily, vitamin D supplements are cheap and readily available. Look for vitamin D3, the form naturally produced by your skin. You can find it in 400, 1,000, and 2,000 IU tablets or capsules. Do not take high doses of vitamin D without your doctor's supervision.

Hungry for another tip? Take your vitamin D supplements with your biggest meal of the day. A recent Cleveland Clinic study found that this strategy increased absorption and boosted blood levels of vitamin D by about 50 percent.

Of course, you can also get your vitamin D from the sun — especially in the summer months. If you're fair-skinned, spending just 10 to 15 minutes in the sun, without sunscreen, should do the trick. If you have darker skin, you can stay in the sun a little longer. Get your dose of sunshine at least twice a week. But don't forget to use sunscreen if you're going to be in the sun longer than 15 to 20 minutes.

Dodge drawbacks of vitamin D

While you probably need more vitamin D, don't go overboard. Taking very high doses over several months could result in vitamin D toxicity. Symptoms include nausea, vomiting, constipation, and weight loss.

High doses of vitamin D can also dangerously increase the calcium levels in your body — and not all of it goes to strengthen your bones. Calcium may be deposited in your kidneys, blood vessels, lungs, and heart. One recent study of black Americans with diabetes linked higher vitamin D levels to calcified atherosclerotic plaque in the aorta and carotid arteries.

You should also be aware of potential drug interactions. Some drugs may deplete or block the absorption of vitamin D. These include corticosteroids, anticonvulsants, and the cholesterol-lowering drug cholestyramine.

Vitamin E

wheat germ • sunflower seeds and oil • safflower oil • almonds • peanuts • spinach • broccoli • fortified margarines and spreads

This fat-soluble nutrient boosts your immune system and widens blood vessels to keep blood from clotting within them. More importantly for your brain, however, vitamin E acts as an antioxidant, guarding cells against damage caused by free radicals. These unstable molecules attack and damage healthy cells in ways that contribute to disease and general aging, a process known as oxidation. Antioxidants disarm free radicals before they do harm.

Vitamin E is not one compound — it's eight, with the most famous being alpha-tocopherol. Supplements sometimes provide only one form of vitamin E, but foods give you a naturally healthy mix. Top-notch sources include wheat germ; sunflower and safflower oils; nuts, especially almonds, peanuts, and hazelnuts; and sunflower seeds.

Not a fan of nuts and seeds? Try second-best sources such as corn oil and soybean oil; green vegetables like spinach and broccoli; and foods fortified with vitamin E like certain breakfast cereals, fruit juices, margarines, and spreads.

You can't get too much vitamin E from foods, but supplements are another story. This nutrient reduces your blood's ability to form clots. Taking high doses of vitamin E supplements boosts your risk of bleeding, particularly of hemorrhagic stroke — serious bleeding in the brain.

Healthy people should not take more than 1,500 International Units (IU) of natural vitamin E or 1,100 IU of synthetic (man-made) vitamin E daily. Older adults may need to set lower limits. Amounts as small as 400 IU a day slightly increased the risk of dying in older adults with existing health problems.

Adults should get 15 milligrams (mg) of vitamin E daily, the equivalent of 22.4 IU. Most people don't. Still, obvious vitamin E deficiencies are rare. They usually only occur in people who can't digest or absorb fat properly, including those with Crohn's disease, cystic fibrosis, and certain rare genetic disorders. Aim to get at least 15 mg of vitamin E daily from food for better brain health.

5 ways vitamin E keeps you sharp

Benefits your blood sugar. Your blood levels of vitamin E may determine your risk of developing diabetes. Getting too few antioxidants, especially vitamin E (alpha-tocopherol) and beta carotene, may play a role in diabetes development.

Research suggests oxidative stress and inflammation contribute to insulin resistance and type 2 diabetes. Oxidative stress occurs when your natural antioxidant defense system gets overwhelmed by free radicals in your body. This imbalance may start before diabetes does, and it may speed up the disease's development.

The oxidative damage done by free radicals may make your cells less sensitive to insulin. Free radicals may also destroy the beta cells in your pancreas that produce insulin. As your blood sugar levels rise, your ability to think quickly and multitask declines. After all, glucose fuels cells. If glucose can't enter your brain cells, they won't have enough energy to function properly. And neurons that aren't working mean a brain that's not working.

Alpha-tocopherol and beta carotene are both powerful antioxidants. Eating enough foods rich in them may soothe oxidative stress and squash inflammation in your body, another predictor of type 2 diabetes.

1 tablespoon wheat germ oil	20.3 mg*
1 oz. dry-roasted almonds	7.4 mg
1 oz. dry-roasted sunflower seeds	6 mg
1 tablespoon sunflower oil	5.6 mg
1 tablespoon safflower oil	4.6 mg
2 tablespoons wheat germ	4 mg
2 tablespoons peanut butter	2.9 mg
1 oz. dry-roasted peanuts	2.2 mg
1/2 cup boiled spinach	1.9 mg
1/2 cup chopped broccoli	1.2 mg

*milligrams

In a study of Swedish men over age 50, those with the lowest amounts of alpha-tocopherol or beta carotene in their blood were the most likely to develop diabetes over the next 20 years. Higher antioxidant levels, however, meant better insulin sensitivity down the road.

Cuts high cholesterol. Eating more vitamin E-rich foods may also improve cholesterol in people with diabetes. Diabetes makes you two to four times more likely to develop heart disease, so controlling your cholesterol becomes especially important.

People with diabetes who ate just under half a cup of whole almonds each day naturally boosted their blood levels of vitamin E, lowered both total and bad LDL cholesterol, and improved their ratio of good HDL cholesterol to bad LDL. All this could add up to a lower risk of heart disease. Munching on almonds also reduced their fasting blood sugar and improved blood sugar control.

Guards against dementia. In a group of men and women over 80 years old, those with the highest levels of vitamin E were about half as likely to develop Alzheimer's disease (AD) over the next six years, compared to those with the least.

Low vitamin E levels may allow beta amyloid deposits to build up in your brain. Mice who had low vitamin E levels and were prone to Alzheimer's made the same amount of beta amyloid as normal mice, but their brains failed to get rid of it effectively.

Fats in your blood help move this substance out of brain cells and into the bloodstream for disposal. Without enough vitamin E, oxidation destroys these hard-working fats. Then beta amyloid builds up, the same way trash does if no one takes it out.

Not all research agrees about the power of vitamin E to guard against Alzheimer's disease. That said, most studies only looked at one form of vitamin E, whereas the newer study in elderly adults measured overall levels of all eight forms of this nutrient.

Don't try to avoid AD by taking supplements. Experts say you're better off getting a balanced mix of vitamin E by eating a variety of foods.

Cushions brain from falls. Falls are the number one cause of traumatic brain injury (TBI) in older adults. People over age 75 have the highest rates of TBI-related hospitalization and death. Having healthy levels of vitamin E in your body before a brain injury could stop you from becoming another statistic. Evidence suggests this nutrient helps protect against brain damage from a TBI.

Brain injuries cause oxidative stress to spike inside your brain, which can harm mental function afterward. Vitamin E neutralizes oxidative stress and counteracts the drop in brain function that happens after a TBI. This nutrient also helps your brain change and adapt after an injury.

Keeps vision clear. People who tend to eat foods high in vitamin E are about 20 percent less likely to develop the blinding disease age-related macular degeneration (AMD). It doesn't take much to reap this protection — just 30 International Units (IU) of vitamin E daily, a little more than the recommended amount.

Vitamin E in combination with other antioxidants may help treat AMD, not just prevent it. A study called AREDS showed that a supplement containing vitamins C and E, beta carotene, zinc, copper, and cupric oxide slowed the progression of AMD and kept it from becoming more advanced. Another supplement, made with vitamins C and E, zinc, lutein, and zeaxanthin, is under study now.

When light enters your eye, it generates free radicals. Over time, the oxidative damage they do to your delicate light-sensing cells may lead to the vision loss of AMD. Scientists think antioxidant nutrients like vitamin E may protect eye cells from the ravages of free radicals.

Supplements aren't the only way to see results. The AREDS study also looked at how many antioxidants people got from food. Those who got the most vitamins C and E, zinc, lutein, zeaxanthin, and omega-3 fats from fish — and ate mostly low-glycemic foods — were the least likely to develop advanced AMD. Low-glycemic foods produce a more gradual rise in blood sugar. Complex carbohydrates, like fiber-rich fruits and vegetables and whole grains, are good choices.

> Foods aren't required to list vitamin E amounts on their Nutrition Facts label unless the food is fortified with it.

Get supplement savvy

You can buy supplements containing natural or man-made vitamin E. The natural form is more potent, so you need less of it. Supplement labels should list synthetic vitamin E as dl-alpha-tocopherol, while natural vitamin E will be listed as d-alpha-tocopherol or "mixed tocopherols." Take them with food, otherwise your body may not absorb this nutrient.

It takes less synthetic vitamin E to cause bleeding problems, compared to the natural form. Avoid taking any vitamin E supplement without your doctor's supervision if you have a vitamin K deficiency, or if you take:

- blood-thinning drugs such as warfarin (Coumadin).

- antiplatelet medications such as clopidogrel (Plavix).

- nonsteroidal anti-inflammatory drugs (NSAIDs) such as ibuprofen or aspirin.

In any case, taking large amounts of alpha-tocopherol, the most common form of vitamin E, may decrease your natural levels of gamma- and delta-tocopherol, other healthy forms of this vitamin. This may do more harm than good.

Some experts recommend you stop using vitamin E supplements about one month before undergoing elective surgery to prevent heavy bleeding.

When vitamin E and exercise don't mix

Taking a combination of 400 International Units (IU) of vitamin E and 1,000 milligrams (mg) of vitamin C supplements daily may cancel out an important benefit of exercise for people who have diabetes.

Becoming more active is one of the best natural treatments for type 2 diabetes, because working muscles improve insulin resistance. But a new exercise study found insulin sensitivity only improved in people not taking these antioxidant supplements.

Exercise naturally generates free radicals inside your body. Normally, that's a bad thing. In this case, however, it's good. Working out only boosts oxidative stress for a short time, not long-term. This quick spike actually helps counteract insulin resistance.

Antioxidant supplements such as vitamins C and E neutralize free radicals. In doing so, they block the temporary oxidation that helps insulin sensitivity and metabolism.

Walking

preserves memory • lowers blood pressure • defends against diabetes • eases stress • battles obesity

"Walking is a man's best medicine," said Hippocrates, the ancient Greek physician and "Father of Medicine." But you may be surprised to learn why he was right.

The occasional evening of lounging in front of the television is all right, but lasting inactivity will wreck a body faster than anything else.

- People who watch four or more hours of television daily were 46 percent more likely to die sooner from any cause, an Australian study found. This may happen because your body changes the way it operates after you have been sedentary for a few hours. For example, an enzyme that removes fat from your blood stops working. That means fat no longer travels to your muscles to be burned as fuel. Instead, it stays in your blood where it can damage your arteries and lead to heart disease.

- People lose about 15 to 25 percent of their brain tissue between ages 30 and 90. But people who exercise regularly lose significantly less, researchers suggest.

- Many diseases of old age have been linked to inflammatory compounds in your body. For example, compounds like interleukin-6, tumor necrosis factor-alpha, and C-reactive protein have been associated with arthritis, heart disease, Alzheimer's disease, age-related macular degeneration, and causes of frailty like sarcopenia — the gradual loss of muscle strength that naturally happens as you grow older. But research shows that walking just 30 minutes a day for five days a week lowers your levels of inflammatory compounds.

- Older adults who participated in a walking program cut their risk of disability by 41 percent, raising their odds of staying independent.

You can see why being sedentary is not as harmless as it seems. But take up walking and you don't have to join a gym — or even break a sweat — to stay healthy. And that's only the beginning. Find out how walking can keep your brain in shape, too.

Grow new brain cells. Once upon a time, doctors thought your brain could not make any new brain cells, but that's not true. Your hippocampus, a part of the brain crucial to learning and memory, can create new brain cells throughout your life. A lot of things determine how many fresh brain cells you can create, but exercise is the strongest generator of new brain cells. Not surprisingly, new brain cells help with learning and memory. In fact, they have been linked to improved brainpower, and they are more likely to be activated when you learn new things.

Make more "brain fertilizer." Exercise triggers your body to produce more of a natural compound called brain-derived neurotrophic factor (BDNF) that can help keep your brain sharp. BDNF helps you form memories, but that's not all. BDNF has been called "brain fertilizer" because it boosts blood flow and neural connections in the brain.

Neural connections are the synapses or links between brain cells. By increasing the number of brain cells and neural connections, some scientists think you build up a savings account of extra neurons and synapses, called cognitive reserve, that protect you against mental decline later in life. This may be one reason why people age 65 and older who walk regularly have a significantly lower risk of vascular dementia, the second most common dementia behind Alzheimer's disease.

Take a "virtual trip" to a scenic location. If you walk with a group and you all use pedometers or know how far you walk, try this. As a group, agree on some interesting locale — such as the Grand Canyon, the Statue of Liberty, or even San Francisco. Set a group goal to walk as many miles as it would take you to get from your town to your chosen spot. Add up everyone's distance totals each week to see how far you've come — and celebrate when you "get there."

Build a bigger brain. Imagine having a younger brain in just six months. It can happen. One sign of aging is the gradual loss of brain volume as decades pass. In other words, your brain shrinks. New research shows that older adults who participated in a walking program for six months increased the size of their brains. In fact, one scientist said their new brain sizes matched the brain volumes of people several years younger. What's more, increases in brain volume are associated with improvements in thinking and remembering. It's like growing smarter as you age.

9 ways walking keeps you sharp

Protects your memory. Walking may be a gentle activity you can do practically anywhere at any time, but don't let that fool you. This easy exercise may still boost your memory, keep your brain from shrinking, and slash your risk of dementia. In fact, this 100-percent natural solution does it all. Just see the evidence for yourself.

- Some people say memory naturally declines with age. But among women age 70 and older, those who regularly walked 1 1/2 hours a week at an easy pace scored higher on memory and thinking tests, a recent study found.

- People over age 65 who walk regularly have less risk of vascular dementia, which is caused by tiny, symptom-free strokes in narrowed arteries. It's the second most common form of dementia after Alzheimer's disease (AD).

- Exercise three or more times a week and you may reduce your risk of dementia by nearly one-third, a study suggests.

- Exercise may be the most powerful trigger for growing new brain cells.

- AD causes the brain to shrink. But a study of people with early Alzheimer's found that those who were more physically fit had less shrinking of the brain than those less fit. That is important because a shrinking brain is associated with poorer thinking and memory. Researchers believe exercises like walking may help preserve more brain cells and prevent shrinking.

Lowers your blood pressure. The next time you are stuck waiting for a prescription or waiting for water to boil, take a 10-minute walk. When people with slightly high blood pressure took just four 10-minute walks a day, they reduced their blood pressure for up to 11 hours afterward.

Experts say regular exercise like walking helps keep your arteries flexible. Because flexible arteries can narrow or dilate as needed, your blood flows easily, and you are less likely to have high blood pressure. This is good news because the Alzheimer's Society reports that people who have high blood pressure are up to 600 percent more likely to develop dementia.

Guards against strokes. People who have had a stroke are 60 percent more likely to develop AD. But women who regularly take brisk walks or who walk for two or more hours a week have at least a 30 percent lower risk of stroke than women who don't walk.

Beats bad cholesterol. You might think you need to "feel the burn" or exercise vigorously to lower your "bad" LDL cholesterol. But a small study of men in their 60s discovered that brisk walking cuts cholesterol, lowers blood pressure, and makes you more physically fit, even if you are already active.

Some studies suggest higher levels of LDL cholesterol may contribute to your risk of vascular dementia. What's more, other studies suggest high LDL may contribute to increasing levels of beta-amyloid, a protein associated with Alzheimer's plaques. More research is needed to determine whether cutting LDL cholesterol helps prevent these dementias. Meanwhile, lowering LDL helps prevent strokes, and avoiding strokes can help prevent dementia.

Add extra steps to your day. Take a 10-minute walk during lunch, use the stairs instead of the elevator, park farther from the store, pace during television commercials, and walk while talking on the phone or waiting for someone.

Soothes stress. Many people treat stress as a natural part of today's busy lifestyle. But stress is a more serious threat than most people think. A 20-year study found that chronic life stress led to a decrease in the volume of the hippocampus, a brain region essential for learning and memory. But experts say exercise can help you shake off the day's tensions, boost the feel-good neurotransmitters in your brain called endorphins, and lower anxiety symptoms. You can even get these results if you are out of shape.

Prevents falls. Falls are the most common cause of brain injury. That is troubling because studies show head injuries raise your risk of both mental decline and dementia. Even worse, one out of every three older adults takes a tumble every year. But you don't have to be one of them. Experts recommend regular exercise to help prevent falls because it builds strength and improves balance. For best results, start with walking and ask your doctor about other exercises that can help.

Trims obesity. Walking can be a great way to lose weight or prevent weight gain. In fact, one study suggests long walks at a slow pace may be a better way to lose weight than faster, shorter walks. Besides, losing weight may help your memory fairly quickly. Here's why. If you are overweight, you are more likely to have higher C-reactive protein levels. High CRP is associated with a less-agile brain. Studies even suggest that weight loss can lead to improvements in memory, especially if you cut calories in addition to walking.

You want to walk regularly but you seem to miss more walks than you take. Here's a great way to fix that problem and have fun doing it. Volunteer to walk dogs at a local shelter, take over the family dog-walking duties, or walk your neighbors' dogs. Research hints that dog walkers exercise more regularly and improve their fitness more than people who walk with a friend.

Fights diabetes. People who walk may cut their diabetes risk by up to 40 percent, according to the Centers for Disease Control and

Prevention. Those who already have diabetes benefit, too. Studies show that exercise can lower blood sugar and improve insulin sensitivity in people with diabetes. This is important because insulin sensitivity problems cause your body to produce too much or too little insulin.

A shortage of insulin affects both diabetes and AD, new research reports. Men who didn't produce the right amount of insulin at age 50 were at a significantly greater risk of developing AD and other dementias later on. Fortunately, just two or three hours of walking a week may make the difference in your diabetes risk and that may slash your dementia risk, as well.

Eases arthritis. Getting arthritis does not mean you have to give up daily walks. In fact, recent research discovered that people who are the least active have 45 percent more risk of dementia than those who are the most active. Besides, experts say gentle exercise, like walking, may actually ease stiffness, make your hips and knees more flexible, and expand your range of motion.

Super secrets of successful walkers

To stay motivated, avoid discomfort, and get the most benefits from your walks, start with these tips.

- Stretch gently for a few minutes before your walk and afterward.

- Stroll slowly for the first five minutes, speed up for the next few minutes, and then walk slowly again for the last five minutes.

- Aim for "moderate intensity" during the speedy part of your walk. You are walking at moderate intensity if you are moving too fast to sing, but you can still talk.

- Add minutes and distance to the fast part of your walk as you become more fit.

- Wear a lightweight, flexible shoe with good cushioning and thick, flexible soles.

- Walk with a buddy or group for safety's sake.

- Buy a pedometer if you need extra motivation to walk. These small devices count the number of steps you take and can use the size of your stride to measure the distance you have walked. For example, 10,000 steps equals roughly five miles. Not only does a pedometer make it easier to set goals and see how you are doing, research also suggests people who use pedometers may walk more every day. You can find reasonably priced pedometers in sporting goods stores.

Walk with peace of mind

Walking should be fun, not risky. Take precautions like these to help you walk without worries.

- Check with your doctor before you begin walking to make sure your health will allow you to walk safely.

- Walk during daylight or in well-lit areas with a buddy and carry your cell phone with you.

- Replace your walking shoes once a year. Frequent use makes the support and cushioning in your shoes wear down enough to raise your risk of injuries.

Water

Water is truly one of your body's natural wonders. It's vital to dozens of different processes and keeps you healthy in hundreds of different ways. This essential substance:

- carries nutrients that keep your cells alive.

- cleans waste material from your tissues and blood.

- lubricates and cushions your joints.

- keeps your digestive system running smoothly.

- maintains your body temperature.

Not surprisingly, nearly all foods contain water. While it is possible to drink too much water, it's a very rare problem, and not one to bother many seniors. After a certain age, you are much more likely to suffer from too little water, or dehydration. That's because you may no longer feel thirst as you used to, so you can actually forget to drink enough.

In addition, an older body doesn't hold onto water the way it once did. If you take certain medications or suffer from certain illnesses — like diabetes, kidney disease, or adrenal gland

You'll get about 1 cup of water from:
1 grapefruit
1 1/2 cups watermelon
1 cup applesauce
2 cups pineapple
1 cucumber
2 cups lettuce plus 1 cup grated carrots
1 cup V8, orange, or apple juice

disorders — your body may dry out faster. Even a sore throat, cold, nausea, or fever makes you less likely to drink as you should.

You can suffer symptoms of mild dehydration after losing less than 5 percent of your body's water weight. Since water makes up about 60 percent of your total weight, a 150-pound person carries about 90 pounds of water. Losing 5 percent of that is equal to 4 1/2 pounds of water. If this happens, you could experience:

- rapid pulse

- low blood pressure

- lack of energy

- decreased mental functioning

- fainting

Here's how drinking just a little water can go a long way to improving your memory and overall brainpower.

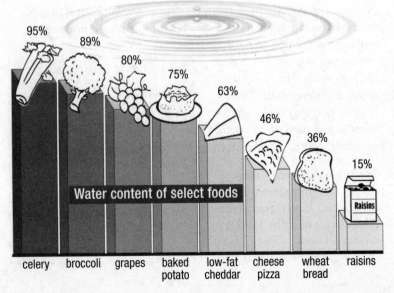

Water content of select foods

95% celery
89% broccoli
80% grapes
75% baked potato
63% low-fat cheddar
46% cheese pizza
36% wheat bread
15% raisins

5 ways water keeps you sharp

Pulls the plug on brain drain. You don't have to drink gallons of water to keep your mind focused and performing. You just don't want to let the water level in your body drop too low. That basically means don't let yourself get dehydrated or your brain will suffer.

While no one gets dehydrated on purpose, it's alarmingly easy to do. Even though losing 5 percent of your water weight is a standard benchmark for dehydration, losing just 2 percent of your body's water weight can affect the way you feel, think, and act. Someone weighing 200 pounds would notice a difference if they lost even 2 1/2 pounds of water.

Tests showed that people suffering this degree of dehydration scored lower on math skills, lost short-term memory abilities, were slower to make decisions, and were generally more fatigued than people with plenty of water to drink.

When you're dehydrated, water moves out of your cells to your bloodstream in an attempt to keep your blood volume and your blood pressure at a safe level. If dehydration continues, your cells shrivel up and no longer work properly. Your brain cells are particularly at risk since your brain is about 70 percent water.

In addition, a lack of adequate water affects your blood brain barrier (BBB). This layer of cells and tissue separates your brain from the rest of your body, protecting it from foreign or dangerous substances in your blood. When you become overheated, without enough fluids to cool your body down, your BBB develops leaks, and that's bad news for your brain function.

Pours on heart-saving power. Strong, steady circulation is key to top-notch brainpower. Your brain cells need the oxygen and nutrients in your blood to do their job and thrive. That's why you want to prevent anything that interrupts or hampers good blood flow.

It may be true that blood is thicker than water, but without enough water, it gets even thicker. Blood is about 78 percent water, so when you get dehydrated, it loses volume. This can cause your blood pressure to drop. It's also more likely to clot now because it's more concentrated. Well-hydrated blood versus dehydrated blood is similar to the difference between potato soup and mashed potatoes. One flows and one doesn't.

> The more water gout sufferers drank, the lower their risk of an attack.

Studies show keeping your body well watered is good for your blood pressure and stroke risk. It may also help avert the dangerous clots that can form in the veins of your legs — a condition called deep vein thrombosis that's common on long flights. That's why airline passengers are urged to drink plenty of water and move around.

Gets tough on gum disease. A beautiful smile means you're taking care of your brain. By making sure you've got healthy teeth and gums you've just taken one risk factor out of the equation for diabetes, heart disease, stroke, and Alzheimer's disease — four conditions that can seriously affect your mental abilities.

Experts believe bacteria in your mouth enter the bloodstream and travel throughout your body causing infection and the inflammation linked to these serious diseases. By eliminating the bacteria, you're removing one spark that can trigger a host of problems.

While brushing, flossing, and regular visits to the dentist are basic to good oral health, a few glasses of water may be the cheapest way to clean your teeth and gums. If you can't brush after each meal, even rinsing your mouth with water can reduce bacteria by 30 percent. Drinking throughout the day triggers your mouth to produce more saliva which, in turn, prevents bacteria and reduces inflammation. This is especially important as you age, since you produce less saliva the older you get.

Drives away diabetes dangers. A few extra glasses of water a day should become part of your regular routine if you suffer from diabetes.

- Substitute water for sugary sodas and other unhealthy drinks and you've taken a big step in controlling your blood sugar levels.

- Water fills you up and could help you eat less, making it easier to drop extra pounds.

- Keeping your body hydrated is important for energy and to help you stay active.

Fends off frightening falls. Major symptoms of dehydration are dizziness, confusion, and low blood pressure. Any of these can cause you to stumble, fall, or faint. A head injury from a fall increases your risk of Alzheimer's disease and other forms of dementia.

A clear look at water filters

Consider getting a home filtration system if clean-tasting, filtered water is important to you but you're stressed out by the bottled water dilemma. Your first step should be determining exactly what contaminants you want to remove from your tap water. Some filtering solutions are designed to do different jobs. Get your water tested then take into account these considerations:

- cost of the initial system

- cost of filter replacements

- the amount of effort required for each type of system

- how much water you use and the speed of filtration

You should then be able to pick out a type or two that fits your requirements — carafe, faucet-mount, countertop, under-sink, reverse-osmosis, or whole-house system. They all have pros and cons, so visit a store where you can get up close and personal with the models, and check out *Consumer Reports* for their own ratings.

Copper causes tap water woes

Look around and chances are you're seeing something that contains copper. The average home contains about 400 pounds of this versatile metal in wiring, electronics, appliances, and water pipes. And that's where a potential problem begins. Long-term exposure to copper in drinking water is linked to memory decline and Alzheimer's disease (AD). Here's what happens.

Water sitting in and flowing through copper pipes gradually absorbs some of the metal. You drink this water and the copper makes its way into your blood-stream and eventually your brain. There it attaches to certain proteins and forms large plaques and tangles that choke off and kill brain cells.

> Call the EPA's Safe Drinking Water Hotline at 800-426-4791 for state-certified testing labs or for your local health authority. They might offer low-cost or free test kits. Or go online at *www. epa.gov/safewater/labs* for your state's contact information.

Multiple studies have shown a definite connection between higher blood levels of copper and lower comprehension scores, memory problems, risk of dementia, and likelihood of AD.

Copper plumbing is used in approximately 90 percent of homes in the United States, and a six-year survey showed more than 4 million people exposed to copper levels over the Environmental Protection Agency limit of 1.3 milligrams per liter. Get your water tested at a state-certified laboratory if you have copper pipes and notice a bitter, metallic taste to your water or blue-green stains on your plumbing fixtures or in your sink. If your copper levels are too high, here's what you can do.

- Replace copper pipes and fixtures with PVC.

- Run water 15 to 30 seconds from every tap before using to flush the copper out.

- Install a home treatment system.

- Use an alternative water source.

Yoga

prevents falls • preserves memory • cuts stress • battles depression • protects your heart • helps you sleep

Imagine an activity that helps your body and mind stay young and vital. You can do it indoors or out, alone or with a group of friends. Best of all, the soothing music and deep breathing help you feel calm and happy.

The activity is yoga, an Indian practice that's more than 5,000 years old. A common form in the West is Hatha yoga, combining physical exercises, breathing techniques, and concentration.

Taking a yoga class with a qualified instructor is a good way to start, since she can explain the movements and correct your posture or help you modify a pose to avoid aggravating an injury. Classes last from 30 to 90 minutes, and you can practice what you learned in class at home. You can also do yoga following an instructional DVD, television show, or iPhone application.

Teaching and certification programs vary widely, but many instructors register with the Yoga Alliance, which has certain minimum requirements. See the Yoga Alliance website at *www.yogaalliance.org* for information about choosing an instructor.

Yoga may look slow and easy, but you'll work your muscles while you move through a series of poses, improving your balance and posture as you practice. It's fairly safe, especially since you can modify the movements and push yourself only as far as feels right.

In addition, yoga isn't a competitive sport. You'll aim to improve, but there's no pressure to "win" a yoga session. And yoga is a lifelong activity you can continue as the years go by.

That makes it an important part of life for someone like Faith, a 55-year-old woman who's been practicing yoga for more than 25 years. She and her doctors credit yoga for her excellent blood pressure and cholesterol readings, along with the healthy bones of a woman decades younger.

Yoga is well-known as a great remedy for arthritis and back pain, but it can also help keep your brain young and agile.

> You may already have a yoga studio at home. You just need a Wii game system, the Wii balance board, and a game that includes yoga. The Wii Yoga game uses the balance board to do yoga, while Wii Fit includes yoga as part of the training.
>
> The balance board gives you instant feedback on your balance and posture — just like a trainer would.

6 ways yoga keeps you sharp

Improves balance to prevent falls. Suffering a fall can mean fractured bones and time in bed — even a slump in brain skills or dementia, including Alzheimer's disease, if you hit your head. But learn the simple motions of yoga, and you'll be able to walk faster, be more flexible, regain your balance, and avoid a dangerous fall.

Researchers at Temple University tested this idea by recruiting older women to do 90 minutes of yoga twice a week for nine weeks. Not only did the women's walking speed and stride length increase, they also enjoyed better posture and balance along with greater leg flexibility. Both the researchers and the women in the study were impressed by how yoga improved their balance and walking.

Keeps your brain young. A workout for your body is also good for your brain. That's because physical exercise boosts blood flow to your brain, delivering the oxygen and glucose brain cells need to live and work. Exercise also encourages your body to produce something called brain-derived neurotrophic factor, a natural chemical that promotes connections between brain cells and helps new cells form.

Studies show staying active can keep your mind sharp as you age. Yoga, blending physical exertion with mental focus, is a powerful brain booster. While you practice yoga postures and pay attention to your breathing and movements, you alter the way you think and perceive the world. Your reaction times become quicker, and your manual dexterity may get better.

Cuts stress. Getting physical causes your body to release endorphins — natural feel-good brain chemicals that help you relax. Yoga is especially powerful, in part because you focus on your breathing and let go of tension.

Researchers in Sweden assigned people to practice yoga and its controlled-breathing methods several times weekly for six weeks. By the end of the study, the yoga participants had less anxiety and stress, along with greater optimism, than a control group that merely sat and relaxed. Because stress leads to inflammation in your body that can eat away at your brain's gray matter, cutting stress is important for keeping your brain healthy.

Beats the blues. Research also shows that people of all ages can practice yoga to reduce depression. Some benefits may come from doing the activity on your own time, gaining a feeling of control. But yoga also gives your brain a boost of the feel-good brain chemical gamma-amino butyric acid (GABA). In fact, yoga is even more effective than a walking program.

A study among women with rheumatoid arthritis found doing yoga three times a week led to less depression along with reduced pain and feelings of disability. Finally, staying social by joining a yoga class may also help you beat the blues.

Protects your heart. Yoga's pattern of deep, slow breathing helps slow your heart rate and lower your blood pressure. Doing yoga also cuts dangerous inflammation in your body while it lowers your level of interleukin-6, a marker for heart disease, stroke, diabetes, and stress. That makes it a great activity to bring down your risk of heart disease.

One study found doing yoga may lead to a healthier heart rhythm among people who practice the activity. Yoga may be an especially good choice if you've already had a stroke. Research shows doing yoga helped people regain their manual dexterity, speaking skills, and balance after a stroke.

Yoga may boost your brain even more than lying quietly with your eyes closed.

Researchers found that men doing a program of yoga poses and guided muscle relaxation for about 25 minutes were more relaxed and better able to concentrate than after they simply lay on their backs. Practicing yoga helped the men feel less anxiety and enjoy a memory boost afterward.

Helps you sleep. Performing yoga along with other relaxation strategies makes a great bedtime routine. You'll put your mind and body in the mood for rest, making it easier to get a good night's sleep. Anything that helps you sleep also helps your brain function.

Yoga for real people

Find a yoga class that fits your needs, no matter your age or health problems. Don't be fooled by the stereotype of young, fit, flexible yoga practitioners. You can find classes designed for people of all ages, sizes, and abilities. Senior centers and retirement communities now host a growing number of gentle yoga classes intended for seniors and people with health or mobility problems. You may even find a class in chair yoga, sitting while you do the movements.

You'll do deep-breathing exercises, practice paying attention to your body, and learn poses that use your arms and legs. This kind of class may work for you if you have balance problems or weak legs, making you shy away from difficult movements, like the warrior or firefly poses. But you'll still work up to being flexible enough to touch your toes or gain enough strength to raise your legs above your waist while sitting.

Doing yoga may help reverse a dowager's hump. Researchers found that seniors with a curve in their upper spine, technically called dorsal kyphosis, enjoyed a small improvement after they attended yoga classes. They did an hour of yoga three times a week for 24 weeks. This study is the first sign that dowager's hump can be improved, and yoga may be the key.

Look for a class with a friendly label like "Gentle Yoga" or "Granny Yoga." If you're really fortunate, you may find an instructor with special certification for teaching seniors, earned from Duke University's Therapeutic Yoga for Seniors program.

Protect fragile eyes

Yoga may not be right for you if you suffer from certain conditions that affect pressure in your eyes. Experts say people who have glaucoma, take anti-glaucoma drugs, or suffer from central retinal vein occlusion, or damage to your retina caused by blocked blood flow, should avoid doing inverted poses — shoulder stands and other positions that keep your head upside down.

You're also at risk if you have a detached retina. These upside-down poses may increase the pressure within your eyeball and damage your vision.

Ask your eye doctor if yoga is safe for your eyes. Also, be sure your yoga teacher is trained and experienced so she can advise you when to avoid a certain pose.

Zinc

oysters • cereal • peanut butter • wheat germ
• veal • seeds • beans • crab • beef

Zinc may be one of the most underappreciated nutrients you'll ever run across. No one goes to the supermarket thinking, "My body needs some extra zinc today." But perhaps you will after you learn about this vital mineral. Even though it's considered a trace element, it's found almost everywhere — in your skin, muscles, bones, and brain. It's not only part of the structure of your body, it helps make important things happen.

You know how striking a match lights a fire? Think of zinc as the spark that lights a match that starts a fire. In this way, zinc is considered a catalyst, because it ignites chemical reactions, mainly through over 100 different enzymes. For example, zinc helps the enzymes that turn carbohydrates, protein, and fat into energy.

6 medium oysters, cooked	76.3 mg
1 cup Total Raisin Bran	15 mg
1 cup canned pork and beans	13.86 mg
3 oz. Alaska king crab	6.48 mg
1 3-oz. hamburger patty	5.36 mg

* milligrams

It's quite common for older adults to have a shortage of zinc. In fact, it can become a vicious cycle. A zinc deficiency dulls your sense of taste and makes you lose your appetite. You don't want to eat, which can make the deficiency worse. In addition, many medications interfere with how well your body absorbs zinc. So even if you're getting enough in your diet, some prescription drugs don't let your body use it.

Possibly the most important thing to remember about zinc is that too much is just as bad as not enough. Too much zinc can be toxic, or poisonous, to nerves, nerve tissues, and cells. This is one supplement you don't want to overindulge in. But don't worry, unless you eat a lot of oysters, it's hard to get more than the upper limit from a healthy diet. The U.S. Food and Nutrition Board says you can safely get up to 40 milligrams (mg) of zinc a day, even though the recommended amount is just 8 to 11 mg.

Zinc deficiency	Zinc overload
Risk of Alzheimer's disease	Risk of Alzheimer's disease
Hormone imbalance	Immune deficiency
Immune deficiency	Cell death
Disrupted thyroid function	Free radical damage
Impaired learning	
Impaired memory	
Damaged neuron function	
Slowed metabolism	
Pain	
Impaired vision	
Cell death	

3 ways zinc keeps you sharp

Helps you think. When experts talk about cognition and cognitive development, they're really talking about fundamental brain skills, like memory, language, thought, attention, and understanding. Zinc's role in all this may not be easy for even scientists to decipher and explain, but they know it's key. They know, for instance, neurons in your brain are full of zinc and that zinc is necessary to move information between them.

Think of it this way. Without communication, not only could you not gossip with your best friend, the world would fall into chaos. The same is true in your body. Your cells absolutely must communicate with each other — this is called cell signaling. Zinc plays a role in this as well as in the process that transmits nerve impulses. Both of these impact everything from learning to building memories.

There are a few other things experts know about zinc and brainpower. If mothers don't get enough when they're pregnant, their babies don't focus or develop as well as others. If children don't get enough during their growing years, they are less able to concentrate and remember. And adults need it to form new nerve cells and protect what's called the blood brain barrier (BBB).

This is a tight layer of cells and tissue that separates your brain from the rest of your body. It keeps potentially damaging substances in your blood, like viruses, from entering your central nervous system — most importantly, your brain. The BBB is especially vulnerable to free radicals, which are unstable molecules that attack normal cells.

Damage from free radicals is called oxidation. When the BBB is oxidized, it allows dangerous substances through. Of course, antioxidants are your body's first line of defense against oxidation, and that's where zinc comes in handy. Its antioxidant powers keep your blood brain barrier strong and leak-free.

Keeps you safe from diabetes. The long-running Nurses' Health Study, funded by the National Institutes of Health, found that women who got the most zinc had about a 20 percent lower risk of developing type 2 diabetes.

There are a couple of proposed ways zinc may help protect you from this devastating disease. Remember, zinc is a catalyst to hundreds of enzyme-related processes, including the creation of insulin. It also has a part in storing insulin and helping it do its job. In addition, because it's an antioxidant, it could protect insulin and cells from attack by free radicals.

If you already get plenty of zinc in your diet, this study showed that taking extra zinc as a supplement didn't give greater protection from diabetes. Supplements were only helpful for those who weren't getting a good amount of zinc from food sources.

Fights the hidden dangers of inflammation. Let's say your sinuses are inflamed. You really feel that pain and pressure in your head. Same with inflamed joints. They ache and maybe even look red. But when there's inflammation in the walls of your arteries, you may never feel a thing.

Doctors can tell, however, because cells in your body produce substances to let other cells know what's going on. One group of substances, inflammatory cytokines, are a red flag that all is not right.

A recent study out of Michigan found that people getting a little extra zinc didn't produce as many inflammatory cytokines as others did, leading the researchers to believe zinc works as an

Phytates are specific compounds found in many high-fiber foods, especially grains and legumes. In your body, they link up with some nutrients — including zinc — and prevent you from absorbing them. Even though some plant foods are good sources of zinc, they aren't as useful as meat sources. Vegetarians should make an effort to get enough zinc from enriched cereals and dairy.

anti-inflammatory. That's powerful natural medicine against all sorts of diseases linked to inflammation, including heart disease and Alzheimer's.

Dodge the dangers of nasal sprays

Zinc has been a popular natural cold remedy for several years because of its antioxidant powers and its ability to help your immune system. You might have bought lozenges, nasal sprays, or nasal gels to help you get over a cold faster. While lozenges are still considered safe, the Food and Drug Administration warned consumers in 2009 to stop using nasal products containing zinc, because some users reported a permanent loss of smell.

> There is a connection between zinc and Alzheimer's disease (AD), but no one agrees whether it is a positive or negative one. Some studies report finding high levels of zinc in brains affected by AD, and say it is partially responsible for amyloid plaques, which form in the brains of Alzheimer's victims. Others say the way zinc protects the blood brain barrier from free radical damage also protects the brain from AD.

Most people don't realize how potentially dangerous this side effect can be. Without a sense of smell, you may not be able to detect a gas leak or smoke. You also won't be able to tell if food is spoiled. While the manufacturers have voluntarily withdrawn these products from stores, you might still have one in your medicine cabinet. Read the labels carefully on nasal sprays and toss any that contain zinc.

Index

A

Abdominal fat 221, 241, 258, 272

Acetaminophen, hearing loss and 131

Acetyl-L-carnitine. *See* L-carnitine

Acupuncture, ringing in your ears and 137

Age-related macular degeneration
blood sugar and 4
dementia and 2
folate and 104
Mediterranean diet and 3
resveratrol and 247
risk factors 2
running and 6
symptoms 1
trans fatty acids and 4
types of 2
vitamin B6 and 317
vitamin E and 337

Aged garlic extract, Alzheimer's disease and 109

Alcohol
caution 250
high blood pressure and 142
sleep and 262

Allergies
gluten 166
quercetin and 99

Alliance of International Aromatherapists 23

Allicin 107

Alpha-linolenic acid (ALA). *See* Omega-3 fatty acids

Alpha-lipoic acid
health benefits 8-10
hearing loss and 134
taking supplements 11

Alpha-tocopherol. *See* Vitamin E

Alzheimer's disease
age-related macular degeneration 2
aged garlic extract and 109
alpha-lipoic acid for 9

apple juice for 97
art therapy for 210
beta carotene for 29
caffeine and 39
calcium and 46
copper plumbing and 352
curcumin and 58
exercise and 242, 342
grape seed extract and 117
green tea and 88
gum disease and 122
head injury and 73
herbal remedies 278
high blood pressure and 139, 322
hypothyroidism and 151
inflammation and 155
L-carnitine for 175
leptin and 217
lowering your risk 18
Mediterranean diet and 228
melatonin supplements and 194
mental exercise and 33-37
music therapy for 204
niacin for 211
obesity and 215
omega-3 fatty acids and 224
plaques, clumps, and tangles 13
resveratrol and 246
risk factors 16
self-tests 20
signs of 12, 15, 17
socialization and 266
stages of 16
standard drug treatments 187
statins and 147
stroke and 144
thiamin deficiency and 306
vitamin B12 and 312
vitamin B6 and 319
vitamin D and 328
vitamin E and 336
walnut extract for 86
zinc and 362

stroke and 292
symptoms 120
water and 350

H